Economic activity and social functioning of adults with psychiatric disorders

Howard Meltzer
Baljit Gill
Mark Petticrew
Kerstin Hinds

London: HMSO

ISBN 0 11 691653 2

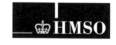

Published by HMSO and available from:

HMSO Publications Centre
(Mail, fax and telephone orders only)
PO Box 276, London SW8 5DT
Telephone orders 0171 873 9090
General enquiries 0171 873 0011
(queuing system in operation for both numbers)
Fax orders 0171 873 8200

HMSO Bookshops
49 High Holborn, London WC1V 6HB
(counter service only)
0171 873 0011 Fax 0171 831 1326
68–69 Bull Street, Birmingham B4 6AD
0121 236 9696   Fax 0121 236 9699
33 Wine Street, Bristol BS1 2BQ
0117 9264306 Fax 0117 9294515
9–21 Princess Street, Manchester M60 8AS
0161 834 7201 Fax 0161 833 0634
16 Arthur Street, Belfast BT1 4GD
01232 238451 Fax 01232 235401
71 Lothian Road, Edinburgh EH3 9AZ
0131 228 4181 Fax 0131 229 2734
The HMSO Oriel Bookshop
The Friary, Cardiff CF1 4AA
01222 395548 Fax 01222 384347

HMSO's Accredited Agents
(see Yellow Pages)

and through good booksellers

Authors' acknowledgements

We would like to thank everybody who contributed to the survey and the production of this report. We were supported by our specialist colleagues in OPCS who carried out the sampling, fieldwork, coding and editing stages.

Great thanks are due to the interviewers who worked on the survey and to the pyschiatrists who conducted the SCAN interviews.

The project was steered by a group comprising the following, to whom thanks are due for assistance and specialist advice at various stages of the survey:

Department of Health:
Dr Rachel Jenkins (chair)
Dr Elaine Gadd
Ms Val Roberts
Ms Antonia Roberts

Psychiatric epidemiologists:
Dr Paul Bebbington
Dr Terry Brugha
Dr Glyn Lewis
Dr Mike Farrell
Dr Jacquie de Alarcon

Office of Population Censuses and Surveys:
Ms Jil Matheson
Dr Howard Meltzer
Ms Baljit Gill
Dr Mark Petticrew
Ms Kerstin Hinds

Most importantly, we would like to thank all the participants in the survey for their time and co-operation.

Contents

Page

Authors' acknowledgements   iii
List of Tables   vii
List of Figures   x
Notes   xii

Focus of the report and survey definitions   xiii

Summary of main findings   xv

1   Economic activity
   1.1   Introduction   1
   1.2   Economic activity and the overall CIS-R score   2
   1.3   Economic activity and neurotic disorders   5
   1.4   Employed people with a neurotic disorder   10
   1.5   Unemployed people with a neurotic disorder   10
   1.6   Finances   10

2   Activities of daily living (ADL)
   2.1   Introduction   29
   2.2   ADL and the overall CIS-R score   29
   2.3   ADL and the neurotic disorders   31
   2.4   Logistic regression   31
   2.5   ADL and specific neurotic disorders   31
   2.6   ADL and the need for help   32

3   Recent stressful life events
   3.1   Introduction   44
   3.2   Stressful life events and CIS-R scores   45
   3.3   Stressful life events and neurotic disorders   46
   3.4   Coping with stressful life events   46
   3.5   Odd ratios of factors associated with having two or more
       stressful life events in the past six months   49

4   Social functioning
   4.1   Introduction   59
   4.2   Perceived social support   59
   4.3   Extent of social networks   60
   4.4   Social and leisure activities   62
   4.5   Relationship between measures of social functioning   63
   4.6   Social functioning and use of services   64

5.   Use of alcohol, drugs and tobacco
   5.1   Alcohol consumption   82
   5.2   Alcohol dependence   85
   5.3   Alcohol problems   88
   5.4   Drug use   90
   5.5   Drug dependence and problems   93
   5.6   Cigarette smoking   95
   5.7   Alcohol consumption, use of drugs and cigarette smoking   97

6 Adults with a psychotic disorder

6.1	Introduction	139
6.2	Descriptive profile	139
6.3	Economic activity	139
6.4	Activities of daily living	140
6.5	Stressful life events	140
6.6	Social functioning	140
6.7	Cigarette smoking, alcohol consumption and drug use	140

7 Adults with suicidal thoughts

7.1	Introduction	147
7.2	Descriptive profile	147
7.3	Economic activity	147
7.4	Activities of daily living	148
7.5	Stressful life events	148
7.6	Social functioning	148
7.7	Cigarette smoking, alcohol consumption and drug use	149

Appendices

A	Psychiatric measurement	
1	Calculation of CIS-R symptom scores	155
2	Algorithms to produce ICD- 10 psychiatric disorders	159
B	Multiple logistic regression (MLR) and odds ratios (OR)	161
Glossary		162

List of tables

Page

Chapter 1: Economic activity
1.1 Economic activity of women and men by CIS-R score (grouped)   11
1.2 Economic activity of women and men by CIS-R score (grouped) and age   12
1.3 Economic activity of women and men by CIS-R score (grouped) and marital status   14
1.4 Economic activity of women and men by CIS-R score (grouped) and qualifications   16
1.5 Economic activity of women and men by CIS-R score (grouped) and non-manual or manual occupation   18
1.6 Economic activity of women and men by CIS-R score (grouped) by physical complaint   20
1.7 Significant Odds ratios associated with the likelihood of not working (compared with working)   22
1.8 Proportions of adults who are permanently unable to work and their characteristcs by CIS-R score   23
1.9 Economic activity by number of disorders by sex   24
1.10 Economic activity of adults with neurotic disorders by sex   25
1.11 Mean number of 'days off work due to ill health' in past year by number of neurotic disorders by sex   26
1.12 Mean number of 'days off work due to ill health' in past year by type of disorder   26
1.13 Behaviour and attitudes of those with a neurotic disorder who were unemployed and seeking work   27
1.14 Receipt of State Benefits   27
1.15 Summary of sources of income   28
1.16 Personal Gross Income   28

Chapter 2: Activities of daily living
2.1 Number of ADL activities by CIS-R score by physical complaint   33
2.2 Type of ADL difficulties by CIS-R score by physical complaint   34
2.3 Number and type of ADL difficulties by number of neurotic disorders by physical complaint   35
2.4 Odds ratios of the correlates of ADL difficulties   36
2.5 Number of ADL difficulties by type of neurotic illness by whether or not has physical complaint   38
2.6 Type of ADL difficulties by type of neurotic illness by physical complaint   39
2.7 Need for help by type of ADL difficulty by neurotic disorder by physical complaint   40
2.8 Type of helper by type of difficulty   43

Chapter 3: Recent stressful life events
3.1 Number of stressful life events experienced in the last six months by CIS-R score and sex   50
3.2 Stressful life events experienced in the last six months by CIS-R score and sex   51
3.3 Number of stressful life events by neurotic disorder   51
3.4 Number of stressful life events by number of neurotic disorders   52
3.5 The proportion of adults with each stressful life event by neurotic disorder   52
3.6 Presence of a neurotic disorder by stressful life events and sex   53
3.7 The receipt of help from family and friends and professionals by stressful life events and the presence or absence of a neurotic disorder   54
3.8 The receipt of professional help by stressful life events and the presence or absence of a neurotic disorder   56
3.9 Odds ratios of neurotic disorder and socio-demographic correlates of having two or more stressful life events   58

Chapter 4: Social functioning
4.1   Perceived social support by age and sex: comparison with Health Survey data   65
4.2   Perceived social support by family unit type and sex   66
4.3   Perceived social support by marital status   66
4.4   Perceived social support by CIS-R score   67
4.5   Perceived social support by neurotic disorder   67
4.6   Perceived social support by number of neurotic disorders   68
4.7   Proportion of adults with a neurotic disorder by perceived social support   68
4.8   Presence of a neurotic disorder by perceived social support and stressful
      life events   68
4.9   Size of primary support group by family unit type and sex   69
4.10 Extent of social networks among those with and without a neurotic disorder   70
4.11 Size of primary support group by CIS-R score and sex   71
4.12 Size of primary support group by neurotic disorder   71
4.13 Size of primary support group by number of neurotic disorders   72
4.14 Proportion of adults with a neurotic disorder by size of primary support group
      and sex   72
4.15 Presence of a neurotic disorder by size of primary support group and stressful
      life events   72
4.16 Odds ratios of neurotic disorder and socio-demographic correlates of having a
      small primary support group (0-3 people)   73
4.17 Odds ratios of neurotic disorder, size of primary support group, and
      socio-demographic correlates of perceiving a severe lack of social support   74
4.18 Participation in leisure activities   75
4.19 Leisure activities by neurotic disorder   76
4.20 Number of leisure activities involved in by CIS-R score and sex   77
4.21 Number of leisure activities involved in by neurotic disorder   77
4.22 Number of leisure activities involved in by number of neurotic disorders   78
4.23 Proportion of adults with a neurotic disorder by number of leisure activities
      involved in   78
4.24 Perceived social support by size of primary support group and sex   78
4.25 Presence of a neurotic disorder by size of primary support group and perceived
      social support   78
4.26 Number of leisure activities involved in by size of primary support group and sex   79
4.27 Presence of a neurotic disorder by size of primary support group and number of
      leisure activities involved in   79
4.28 Number of leisure activities involved in by perceived social support and sex   80
4.29 Presence of a neurotic disorder by perceived social support and number of
      leisure activities involved in   80
4.30 Receipt of services by level of perceived social support   81

Chapter 5: Use of alcohol, drugs and tobacco
5.1   Alcohol consumption level by sex: a comparison with the 1993 Health Survey   99
5.2   Alcohol consumption level by age (grouped) and sex   100
5.3   Alcohol consumption level by CIS-R score (grouped) and sex   101
5.4   Alcohol consumption level by neurotic disorder and sex   102
5.5   Alcohol consumption level by type of neurotic disorder and sex   103
5.6   Alcohol consumption level by number of neurotic disorders and sex   104
5.7   Significant odds ratios associated with alcohol consumption a) of less than 1 unit
      per week and b) of more than 35 units (women) or 50 units (men) per week   105
5.8   Neurotic disorder by alcohol consumption level and sex   106
5.9   Reasons for not drinking alcohol by whether subject has always been a non-drinker
      or has stopped drinking and neurotic disorder   106

5.10 Alcohol dependence by alcohol consumption level and sex   107
5.11 Alcohol dependence by age (grouped) and sex   108
5.12 Alcohol dependence by CIS-R score (grouped) and sex   109
5.13 Alcohol dependence by neurotic disorder and sex   109
5.14 Alcohol dependence by the number of neurotic disorders and sex   110
5.15 Alcohol dependence by neurotic disorder, alcohol consumption level and sex 110
5.16 Significant odds ratios associated with being alcohol dependent (compared with
      not being dependent)   111
5.17 Prevalence of neurotic disorder by alcohol dependence and sex   112
5.18 Alcohol problems by consumption level and sex   113
5.19 Alcohol problems by CIS-R score (grouped) and sex   114
5.20 Alcohol problems by neurotic disorder, consumption level and sex   115
5.21 Alcohol problems by the number of neurotic disorders and sex   116
5.22 Significant odds ratios associated with having an alcohol problem (compared
      with not having a problem)   117
5.23 Prevalence of neurotic disorder by type of alcohol problem and sex   118
5.24 Percentage of adults having an alcohol problem by neurotic disorder, alcohol
      dependence and sex   118
5.25 Use of drugs by sex: all adults   119
5.26 Use of drugs by age and sex   120
5.27 Use of drugs by sex: adults who took drugs   121
5.28 Percentage of adults taking each drug type who also took another type of drug 121
5.29 Use of drugs (grouped) by CIS-R score(grouped) and sex   122
5.30 Use of drugs (grouped) by type of disorder and sex   123
5.31 Use of drugs (grouped) by the number of neurotic disorders and sex   124
5.32 Significant odds ratios associated with drug use (compared with no drug use) 125
5.33 Prevalence of neurotic disorder by the use of drugs by sex   126
5.34 Drug dependence and problems by sex and by age (grouped)   126
5.35 Drug dependence and drug problems by neurotic disorder and sex   127
5.36 Drug dependence (related to the type(s) of drug taken) and neurotic disorder
      by the type of drug   127
5.37 Significant odds ratios associated with being drug dependent (compared with not
      being dependent)   128
5.38 Significant odds ratios associated with having a drug problem (compared with
      having no problem)   129
5.39 Sex, age, and the number of neurotic disorders by the use of drugs, dependence
      and problems   130
5.40 Cigarette smoking by sex: a comparison with the 1993 Health Survey   131
5.41 Cigarette smoking by age (grouped)   132
5.42 Cigarette smoking by CIS-R score (grouped) and sex   133
5.43 Cigarette smoking by type of neurotic disorder and sex   134
5.44 Cigarette smoking by the number of neurotic disorders and sex   134
5.45 Significant odds ratios associated with cigarette smoking (compared with not
      smoking cigarettes)   135
5.46 Prevalence of neurotic disorder by cigarette smoking and sex   136
5.47 Cigarette smoking and drug use by alcohol consumption level and neurotic
      disorder   136
5.48 Alcohol consumption level and cigarette smoking by the use of drugs and
      neurotic disorder   137
5.49 Alcohol consumption level and drug use by cigarette smoking and neurotic
      disorder   137
5.50 Significant odds ratios associated with neurotic disorder (compared with no
      neurotic disorder)   138

Chapter 6: Adults with a psychotic disorder

6.1 Economic activity of adults with (a) a psychotic disorder, (b) a neurotic
disorder and (c) no psychiatric disorder   142

6.2 Financial situation of adults with (a) a psychotic disorder, (b) a neurotic
disorder and (c) no psychiatric disorder   142

6.3 Difficulties with ADL of adults with (a) a psychotic disorder, (b) a neurotic
disorder and (c) no psychiatric disorder   143

6.4 Stressful life events of adults with (a) a psychotic disorder, (b) a neurotic disorder
and (c) no psychiatric disorder   144

6.5 Size of primary support group and degree of perceived social support for adults
with (a) a psychotic disorder, (b) a neurotic disorder and (c) no psychiatric disorder   144

6.6 Participation in outdoor and indoor leisure activities for adults with (a) a psychotic
disorder, (b) a neurotic disorder and (c) no psychiatric disorder   145

6.7 Attendance at social, training or educational centres of adults with (a) a psychotic
disorder (b) a neurotic disorder and (c) no psychiatric disorder   146

6.8 Use of tobacco, alcohol and drugs for adults with (a) a psychotic disorder
(b) a neurotic disorder and (c) no psychiatric disorder   146

Chapter 7: Adults with suicidal thoughts

7.1 Economic activity of adults with suicidal thoughts compared with those with a
neurotic disorder and those with no psychiatric disorder   150

7.2 Financial situation of adults with suicidal thoughts compared with those with a
neurotic disorder and the general population   150

7.3 Difficulties with ADL of adults with suicidal thoughts compared with those with
a neurotic disorder and those with no psychiatric disorder   151

7.4 Stressful life events of adults with suicidal thoughts compared with those with a
neurotic disorder and those with no psychiatric disorder   152

7.5 Size of primary support group and degree of perceived social support for adults
with suicidal thoughts compared with those with a neurotic disorder and no
psychiatric disorder   152

7.6 Participation in leisure activities for adults with suicidal thoughts compared with
those with a neurotic disorder and those with no psychiatric disorder   153

7.7 Attendance at social, training or educational centres of adults with suicidal
thoughts compared with those with a neurotic disorder and those with no
psychiatric disorder   154

7.8 Use of tobacco, alcohol and drugs by those with suicidal thoughts compared with
those with a neurotic disorder and those with no psychiatric disorder   154

List of figures

Chapter 1: Economic activity

1.1 Economic activity by CIS-R score: Women   2

1.2 Economic activity by CIS-R score: Men   3

1.3 Proportion of adults working by CIS-R score by age   4

1.4 Proportion of adults working by CIS-R score by marital status   6

1.5 Proportion of adults working by CIS-R score by qualifications   7

1.6 Proportion of adults working by CIS-R score by social class   8

1.7 Proportion of adults working by CIS-R score by physical complaints   9

Chapter 2: Activities of daily living
2.1   Proportion of adults with any ADL difficulty by CIS-R score (grouped) by sex   30

Chapter 3: Recent, stressful life events
3.1   Number of stressful life events in past 6 months by CIS-R score   45
3.2   Stressful life events strongly associated with neurotic disorders   47
3.3   Proportion of adults with a neurotic disorder by stressful life event   48

Chapter 5: Use of alcohol, drugs and tobacco
5.1   Multiplying factors for converting drinking frequency and number of units
       consumed on a usual day into a number of units consumed each week   84
5.2   Alcohol consumption categories, based on usual weekly consumption (units) over
       the previous 12 months   87
5.3   Criteria for the definition of alcohol dependence   96

Notes

1 Tables showing percentages

The row or column percentages may add to 99% or 101% because of rounding.

The varying positions of the percentage signs and bases in the tables denote the presentation of different types of information. Where there is a percentage sign at the head of a column and the base at the foot, the whole distribution is presented and the individual percentages add to between 99% and 101%. Where there is no percentage sign in the table and a note above the figures, the figures refer to the proportion of people who had the attribute being discussed, and the complementary proportion, to add to 100%, is not shown in the table.

Standard errors are shown in brackets beside percentages in the tables.

The following conventions have been used within tables showing percentages:

-	no cases
0	values less than 0.5%

2 Small bases

Very small bases have been avoided wherever possible because of the relatively high sampling errors that attach to small numbers. Often where the numbers are not large enough to justify the use of all categories, classifications have been condensed. However, an item within a classification is occasionally shown separately, even though the base is small, because to combine it with another large category would detract from the value of the larger category. In general, percentage distributions are shown if the base is 30 or more. Where the base is slightly lower, actual numbers are shown in square brackets

3 Significant differences

The bases for some sub-groups presented in the tables were small such that the standard errors around estimates for these groups are biased. Confidence intervals which take account of these biased standard errors were calculated and, although they are not presented in the tables, they were used in testing for statistically significant differences. Statistical significance is explained in Appendix B to this Report.

Focus of the report and survey definitions

Focus of the Report

This report is one of three looking at data from the private household survey of the OPCS surveys of psychiatric morbidity. The report focuses mainly on the economic and social functioning of those with neurotic disorders[1]. A separate chapter is devoted to the small group of people with psychotic disorders.

More specifically, this report covers the following topics

- economic activity
- financial circumstances (receipt of State Benefits, sources of income and gross, individual income)
- difficulties with activities of daily living (ADL) and the help needed and received among those experiencing difficulty
- experience of recent stressful life events and coping strategies
- the extent of social support from family and friends
- participation in 'home based' and 'out of the home' social activities
- cigarette smoking, alcohol consumption, drug use and its consequences

The first five chapters of this report focus on the extent to which people with neurotic disorders differ from those without a neurotic disorder on various measures of economic and social functioning and investigate differences between those with different neurotic disorders.

Because data on many of the topics covered in this report were collected for all respondents, just over 10,000, analysis has been carried out by CIS-R scores as well as by type of neurotic disorder[2]. Results of the CIS-R analysis are included in this Report as they allow a more detailed examination of those whose neurotic

symptomatology is at a level below that classifiable as a neurotic disorder

Two relatively small groups of survey respondents, those classified as having a psychotic disorder (44 adults) and those with suicidal thoughts (80 adults) have been allocated a chapter each: Chapters 6 and 7 respectively.

Other reports on the private household survey

Report 1

Report 1, published in Spring 1995, details the prevalence of neurotic symptoms and neurotic and psychotic disorders in the general population. It shows that prevalence of symptoms and disorders varied according to a number of personal, social, and economic characteristics, such as sex, family unit type, and working status. Report 1 also shows the prevalence of alcohol and drug dependence.

Some findings from Report 1

- Compared with those working full time, the odds of having most neurotic disorders were more than doubled among unemployed and economically active people.

- Age was particularly associated with alcohol and drug dependence, with the odds of having these disorders decreasing with age

Report 1 also includes information on the survey methodology: the sample design, response, and the method used to weight the data. The questionnaires used in the survey are printed as an Appendix to Report 1.

Report 2

The topics covered in Report 2 are physical complaints, the use of services and receipt of treatment for adults with psychiatric disorders. The format is similar to this report in that the last two chapters focus on those with psychotic disorders and suicidal thoughts respectively.

Survey definitions

The measures of psychiatric morbidity used in this Report

Ten neurotic disorders are identified in this report. They are:

- mixed anxiety and depressive disorder
- generalised anxiety disorder
- mild, moderate and severe depressive episode (collectively grouped as depressive episode for many analyses)
- agoraphobia, social phobia and specific isolated phobia (individuals could only have one of these and they are combined as 'phobia' for much analysis)
- Obsessive-Compulsive Disorder
- panic disorder

The way in which each of these disorders was identified is shown in Appendix A. It is worth noting here that mixed anxiety and depressive disorder was a catch-all category for adults with a neurotic disorder who failed to meet the research diagnostic criteria for one of the other nine disorders identified. This means that while people could have more than one of the other disorders, mixed anxiety and depression was only ever present on its own.

The chapter on psychotic disorders groups together all adults found to have any psychotic illness as prevalence of these disorders was very low. The way in which psychotic disorders were identified is shown in Appendix A.

When looking at neurotic disorders in this Report, every individual with each disorder is included in order to understand the associations with social, economic and lifestyle characteristics. This differs from the use of the primary disorder hierarchy used in Report 1 to produce prevalence estimates[3]. Those with a psychotic disorder are excluded from the chapters covering neurotic disorders.

This report presents no information about the 316 interviews conducted by proxy as neurotic diagnoses could not be obtained for this group.

Notes and references

1   The private household survey involved interviews with 10,000 randomly sampled adults in Great Britain. In addition to the private household survey, interviews were also conducted in institutions specifically catering for people with mental illness and among the homeless.

2   Lewis, G. and Pelosi, A. J., *Manual of the Revised Clinical Interview Schedule, (CIS-R)*, June 1990, Institute of Psychiatry.

Lewis, G., Pelosi, A.J., Araya, R.C. and Dunn, G., (1992) Measuring Psychiatric disorder in the community: a standardized assessment for use by lay interviewers, *Psychological Medicine*, **22**, 465-486

The CIS-R was an instrument used to measure neurotic psychopathology. More information about the CIS-R is included in Appendix A.

3   In Report 1 individuals were classified according to their most severe or primary disorder. The disorder hierarchy used to identify primary disorders is shown in Appendix A of this report.

Summary of main findings

The findings described in this report and summarised here focus on the associations between having a neurotic disorder and measures of economic activity and social functioning for people aged 16 to 64. Causal relationships should not be assumed for any of the results presented in this report.

Economic activity (Chapter 1)

- Adults with neurotic health problems were four to five times more likely than the rest of the sample to be permanently unable to work.

- Among women with a phobia, only 3 in 10 were working; among men, 4 in 10.

- Those with two or more neurotic disorders who had been working for at least one year had on average 28 days a year off sick compared with 8 days a year for those with one neurotic disorder.

- Among the sample with any neurotic disorder who were unemployed and seeking work, 70% had been unemployed for a year or more, that is, approximately 7% of all people with a neurotic disorder.

- Compared with the general population, adults with neurosis were twice as likely to be receiving Income Support (19% compared to 10%) and four to five times more likely to be on Invalidity Benefit (9% compared to 2%).

- The median, weekly, gross income among those with a neurotic disorder was about £90 compared with £150 for the general population.

Activities of Daily Living - ADL
(Chapter 2)

- Among adults reporting no physical health problem, 35% of those with two neurotic disorders had at least one ADL difficulty, practically twice the proportion of those with one neurotic disorder (19%), and over four times the proportion without a neurotic disorder (8%).

- People with phobia, depressive episode and Obsessive-Compulsive Disorder (OCD) had the highest proportions with any ADL difficulty, 55%, 45% and 42%.

- Between 10 and 20 percent of adults with generalised anxiety disorder (GAD), depressive episode, phobias or OCD experienced difficulty with managing money or dealing with paperwork.

Recent stressful life events (Chapter 3)

- Seventy one percent of adults with a neurotic disorder had experienced one of the 11 stressful life events measured by the survey in the previous 6 months compared with 48% of those with no disorder.

- 26% of women and 18% of men with any stressful life event had a neurotic disorder compared with 13% and 7% respectively of those with no stressful life events.

- Stressful life events strongly associated with having a neurotic disorder were: problems with the police, a serious problem with a close friend, and a financial crisis; over a third of people experiencing each of these events had a neurotic disorder.

Social functioning (Chapter 4)

- The prevalence of neurotic disorder among adults with a severe lack of social support (29%), was double that of adults with no such lack (14%).

- Adults with phobia and depressive episode were most likely to report a lack of social support; over half felt some lack of social support compared with a third of those with no neurotic disorder.

- One fifth of those with phobia, depressive episode and Obsessive-Compulsive Disorder had a particularly small circle of family or friends (less than 4 adults) giving support, compared with only 6% among those with no neurotic disorder

- One in five adults with depressive episode participated in less than 4 leisure activities compared with one in 20 of those with no neurotic disorder

Use of alcohol, drugs and tobacco (Chapter 5)

- Adults with a neurotic disorder were more likely than those without disorder to:

  - abstain from drinking alcohol or drink less often than once a week (26% compared with 19%). Men with neurosis were also more likely to drink over the recommended safe maximum of 50 units a week (12%) than those with no disorder (7%).

  - have used drugs in the past year, including the misuse of prescribed medicines (10% compared with 4%).

  - smoke cigarettes (44% compared with 29%) as well as to smoke heavily (18% compared with 10%)

- Among regular drinkers, alcohol dependence was more than twice as common

among those with a neurotic disorder (12%) than those with no such disorder (5%).

- Similarly, regular drinkers with a neurotic disorder were more likely to have experienced an alcohol-related problem in the past year (22%) than those without a neurotic disorder (14%).

- Drug dependence was twice as common among drug takers with a neurotic disorder (60%) than among those with no such disorder (32%).

- Drug takers with a neurotic disorder were more likely to have experienced a drug-related problem (36%) than those who had no such disorder (20%).

Adults with a psychotic disorder (Chapter 6)

- Only 4 in 10 adults with a psychotic disorder were working compared with nearly 6 in 10 of those with a neurotic disorder and 7 in 10 of those unaffected by a mental disorder.

- The median, weekly, gross, individual income of the group with psychosis was £90 compared with £150 for those without a psychiatric disorder.

- Among those with psychoses, 22% had difficulty managing money such as budgeting for food or paying bills.

- 54% of people with psychosis felt a moderate or severe lack of social support compared with 45% of people with neurosis and 36% of those with no psychiatric disorder.

- Ten percent of the adults with psychosis went to a 'club for people with mental health problems' and 5% attended 'a Day Centre for social reasons'.

- Those with a psychotic disorder were about twice as likely as those with a neurotic disorder to have used cannabis in the past year (16% compared with 9%) who in turn were twice as likely as those with no disorder to have used this drug (9% compared with 4%).

Adults with suicidal thoughts
(Chapter 7)

Only those with significant depressive symptoms in terms of frequency, severity, or duration were also asked questions relating to depressive ideas including suicidal thoughts. Thus, people with suicidal thoughts who did not have significant depressive symptoms are not included in the analysis.

- Only about a quarter of adults with suicidal thoughts were working compared with just over a half of those with any neurotic disorder and about three-quarters of those with no psychiatric problem

- Compared with the sample unaffected by psychiatric problems, those with suicidal thoughts were four times more likely to be in receipt of Income Support (40% compared with 10%) and seven times more likely to be on Invalidity Benefit (14% compared with 2%)

- Among those with suicidal thoughts, a half had difficulty with at least one activity of daily living compared with a third of those with a neurotic disorder and an eighth of those without a psychiatric disorder.

- 85% of those with suicidal thoughts had at least one stressful life event in the 6 months prior to interview; among the no disorder group, 48% had experienced at least one event.

- 43% of the group with suicidal thoughts felt a severe lack of social support compared with 17% of those with any neurotic disorder and 8% of those with no psychiatric disorder.

- Among those with thoughts of killing themselves, 52% were smokers compared with 30% of the no disorder group. Furthermore, among those with suicidal thoughts who smoked, 44% were heavy smokers compared with 33% of smokers with no psychiatric disorder

1 Economic activity

1.1 Introduction

In Report 1, the prevalence of neurotic health problems, symptoms and disorders were presented by employment status: working full time, part time, unemployed or economically inactive.[1] In this Report, we examine variations in economic activity, rather than employment status, among those with neurotic disorders. The relationship between economic activity and employment status is shown in the illustration below: economic activity has a more detailed categorisation of those who were not in paid employment in the week prior to interview.

In this chapter, we also take a special look at topics relevant to employed and unemployed adults who had a neurotic disorder. For those who were employed, time off work due to illness is investigated. Four issues are explored for the unemployed group: length of time unemployed; whether a mental health problem was cited as a cause of their unemployment; job seeking behaviour; and the extent to which mental health problems were felt to cause difficulties in finding new employment.

Finally in this chapter, some aspects of the financial circumstances of people with a neurotic disorder are examined.

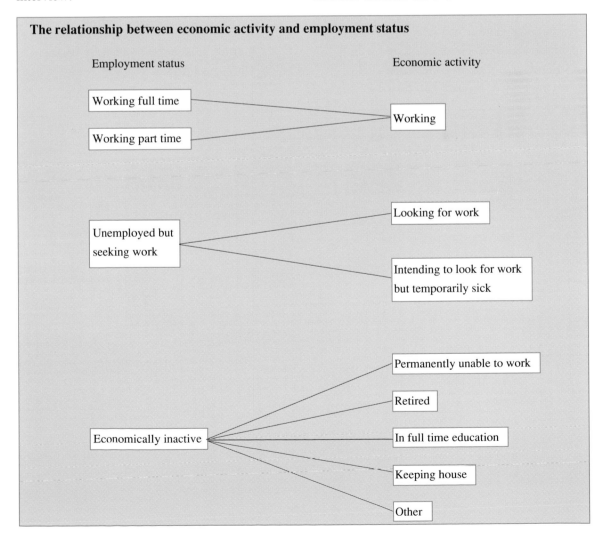

The relationship between economic activity and employment status

1.2 Economic activity and the overall CIS-R score

Among the whole population, economic activity is not only affected by sex but by many other factors including age, marital status, educational attainment, social class and the existence of a limiting longstanding illness.[2] These five factors are also related to each other. Thus, Tables 1.1 to 1.6 which show the distribution of economic activity of men and women by CIS-R groups for each factor separately, are confounded by the presence of the others. The results from logistic regression analysis which looks at the association between neurotic disorders and economic activity controlling for other factors are presented in Table 1.7. The crosstabulations and their diagrammatical representations are presented here initially for descriptive purposes.

For both men and women, there were clear patterns of differences in economic activity by CIS-R scores. *(Figure 1.1 & Table 1.1)*

- The proportions of men and women who were working decreased with increasing CIS-R scores: from 78% to 51% among men and from 66% to 48% among women.

- The proportions of men and women looking for work were significantly larger among those with CIS-R scores of 12 or more: twice as large for women and one and a half times larger for men.

- The most marked difference among CIS-R groups was in the proportions who were classified as permanently unable to work. Those with a score of 18 or higher were three to five times more likely to be permanently unable to work than the population average: 24% compared with 5% among men and 11% compared with 3% among women.

- About a fifth of all women were 'keeping house'. This proportion hardly varied within each CIS-R group.

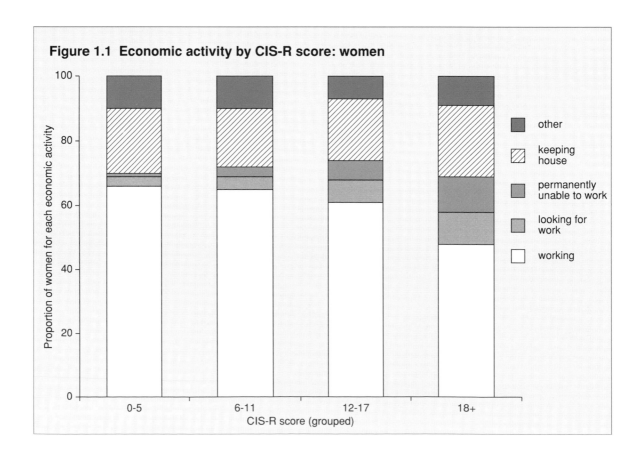

Figure 1.1 Economic activity by CIS-R score: women

Age

When age and sex were examined together, the largest disparity in the distribution of economic activity among CIS-R groups was found among those aged 40-64, particularly for men. *(Figure 1.2 & Table 1.2)*

Men aged 40-64 with a CIS-R score of below 6 were twice as likely to be working compared with their equivalents who had a score of 18+ (77% compared with 38%). In these same two CIS-R groups 5% and 45% respectively were permanently unable to work.

The most conspicuous difference in economic activity between the two age groups, 16-39 and 40-64 was among men with a CIS-R score of

18+: 63% of the younger group were working compared with 38% of the older men. Conversely, 45% of the older group were permanently unable to work compared with 4% of the those aged 16-39.

Marital status

Given the overall trend of a decrease in the proportion of people working as the CIS-R score increases, differences in economic activity by marital status show a consistent pattern. Within each CIS-R group, for both men and women, higher proportions of those who were married or cohabiting were working compared with those who were single or had been married. *(Figure 1.3 and Table 1.3)*

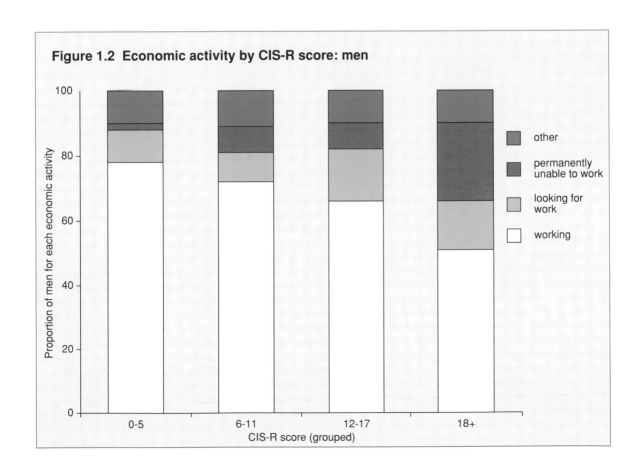

Figure 1.2 Economic activity by CIS-R score: men

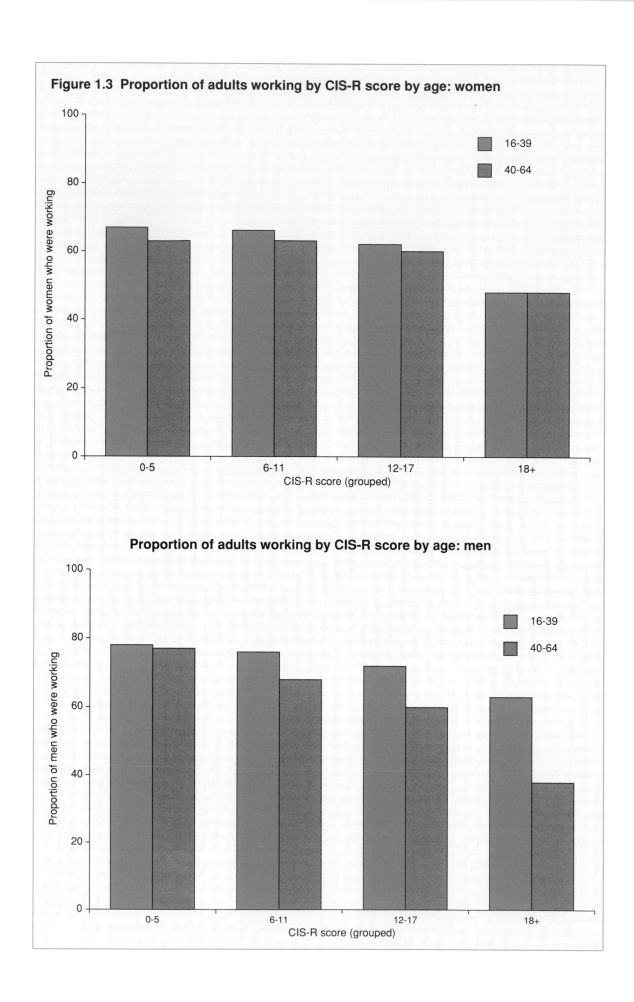

Figure 1.3 Proportion of adults working by CIS-R score by age: women

Proportion of adults working by CIS-R score by age: men

Educational attainment

Educational attainment is summarised in terms of whether or not the respondent had formal qualifications. As would be expected those with qualifications were far more likely to be working than those who had finished their full time education without any qualifications. However, Figure 1.4 shows that there is a strong interaction between CIS-R scores and educational attainment in relation to economic activity, particularly among men. Around two-thirds of men without qualifications with a score below 6 on the CIS-R were working compared with a quarter of unqualified men who had the highest CIS-R scores. It is a remarkable statistic that nearly half the men, without qualifications in the 18 plus CIS-R group were permanently unable to work. Looking at women, the CIS-R score seems to have a lesser effect. *(Figure 1.4 and Table 1.4)*

Social class

The distribution of economic activity by CIS-R according to social class is similar to that for qualifications though the differences in economic activity between those in manual and non-manual were less pronounced. The reason for this is that those in non-manual occupations were more likely to have qualifications than those in manual jobs. *(Figure 1.5 and Table 1.5)*

Physical illness

The group of adults who had a combination of a physical illness and a neurotic health problem, especially with a score of 18 plus on the CIS-R, tended to have the smallest proportion who were working (42% of women and 38% of men) and the largest proportion of those permanently unable to work (18% of women and 37% of men) compared with any other group. *(Table 1.6 and Figure 1.6)*

The relative contribution of factors associated with economic activity

Logistic regression analysis was used to quantify the increase in odds of not-working compared to working associated with a neurotic health problem, ie having a score of 12 or more on the CIS-R. Table 1.7 demonstrates very clearly that many factors were associated with increasing odds of not working compared with working: being a woman, belonging to an ethnic minority, being a single parent, living in rented accommodation, being in social class III non-Manual, IV or V; having no qualifications, being aged 55-64, and having a physical illness. Controlling for all the factors, a neurotic health problem increased the odds ratio of not working to working by about fifty percent, the same increase as that for having a physical illness. *(Table 1.7)*

Another way of showing how the relationship between CIS-R scores and economic activity is affected by other factors is by looking at inter-action effects. In Table 1.8, the focus of attention are those permanently unable to work. Even though a combination of sex, age and social class was a major factor governing economic activity, adults with neurotic health problems (a CIS-R score of 12 or more) were four to five times more likely than the rest of the sample to be permanently unable to work. *(Table 1.8)*

1.3 Economic activity and neurotic disorders

There were significant differences in economic activity between those with one, and two or more neurotic disorders. Both men and women with comorbid neurotic disorders were less likely to be working, and more likely to be permanently unable to work compared with those with one neurotic disorder. *(Table 1.9)*

Looking at the particular neurotic disorders, people with phobias stand out from the rest in that only 3 in 10 women were working; among men, 4 in 10. For both men and women with phobic disorders, about a quarter were looking for work or would look if not temporarily sick and a fifth were permanently unable to work. *(Table 1.10)*

Figure 1.4 Proportion of adults working by CIS-R score by marital status: women

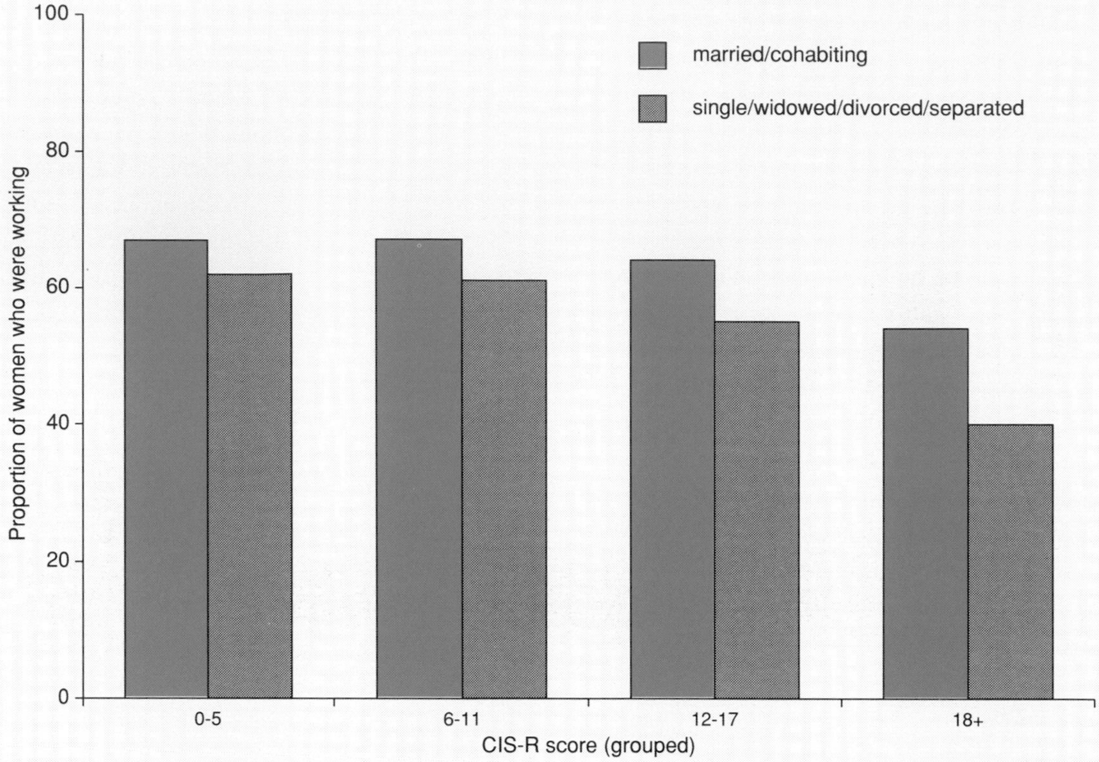

Proportion of adults working by CIS-R score by marital status: men

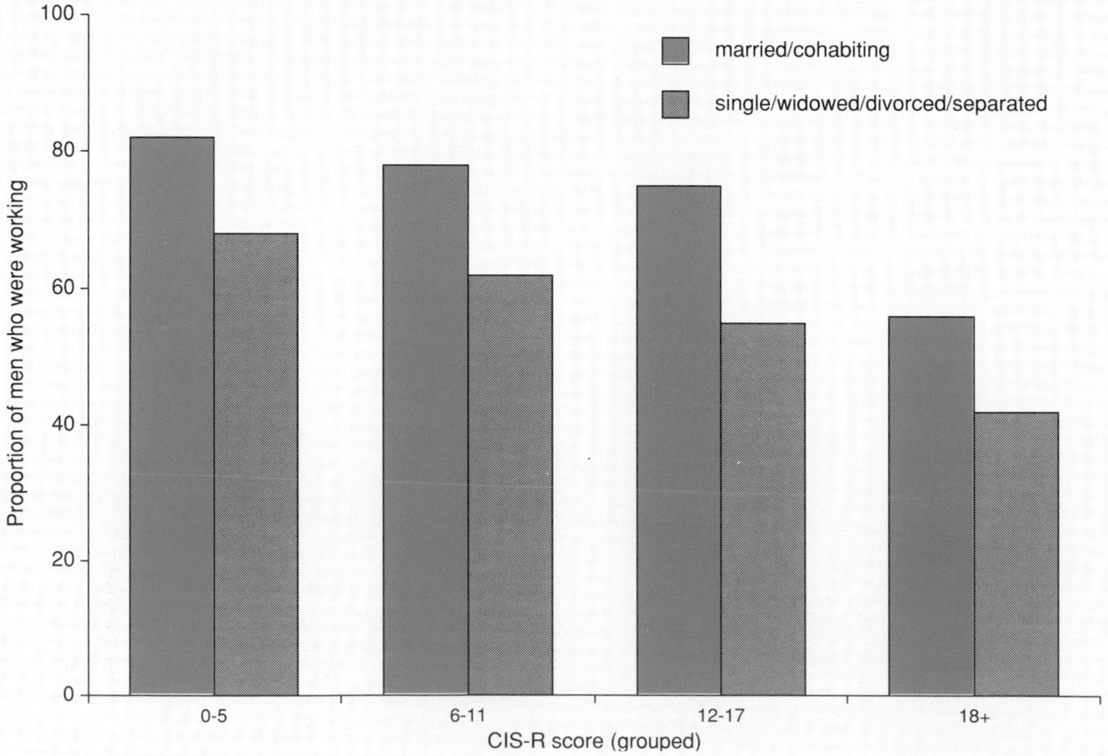

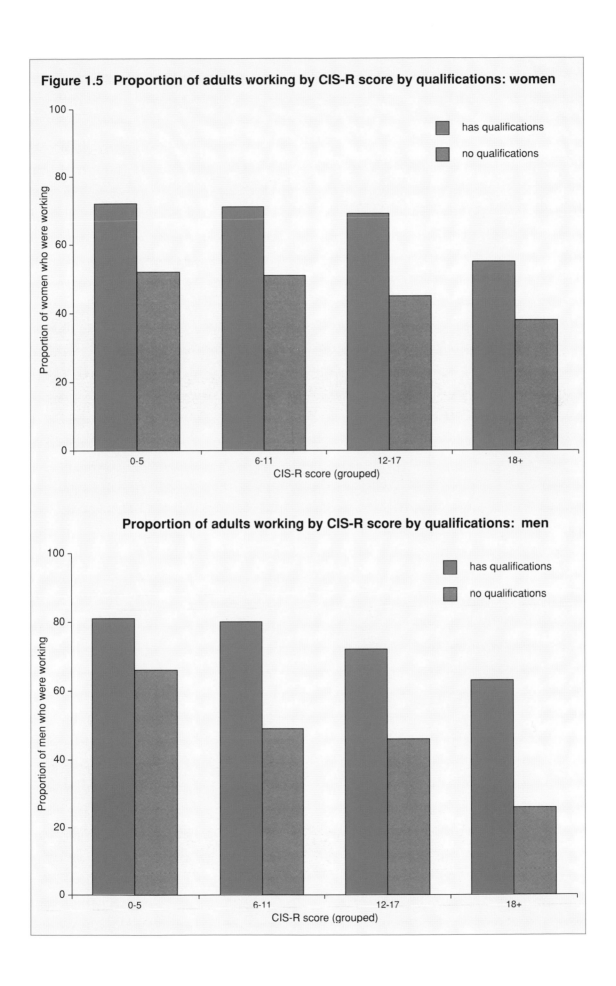

Figure 1.5 Proportion of adults working by CIS-R score by qualifications: women

Proportion of adults working by CIS-R score by qualifications: men

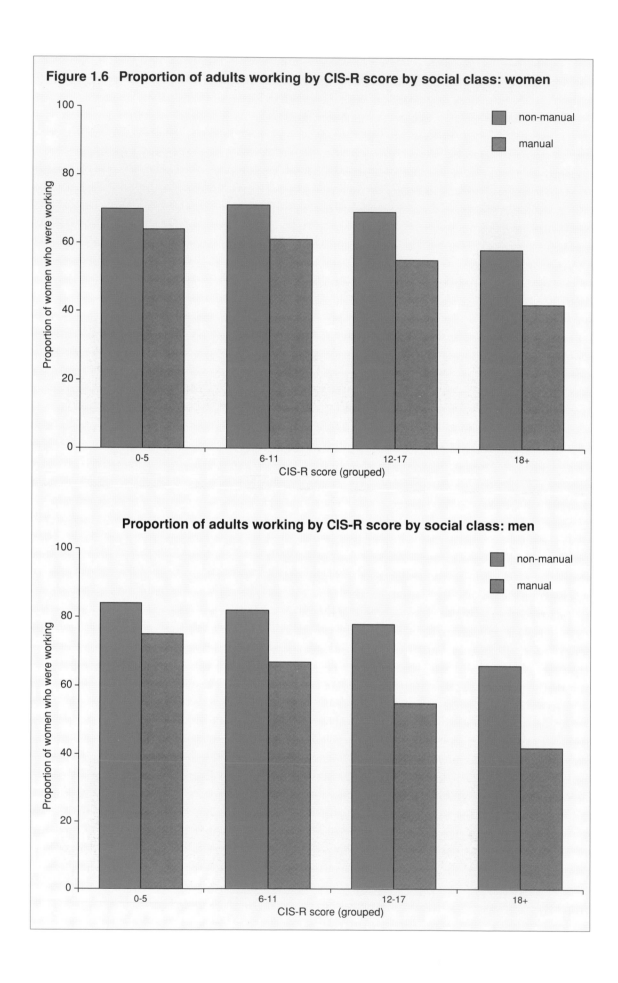

Figure 1.6   Proportion of adults working by CIS-R score by social class: women

Proportion of adults working by CIS-R score by social class: men

8

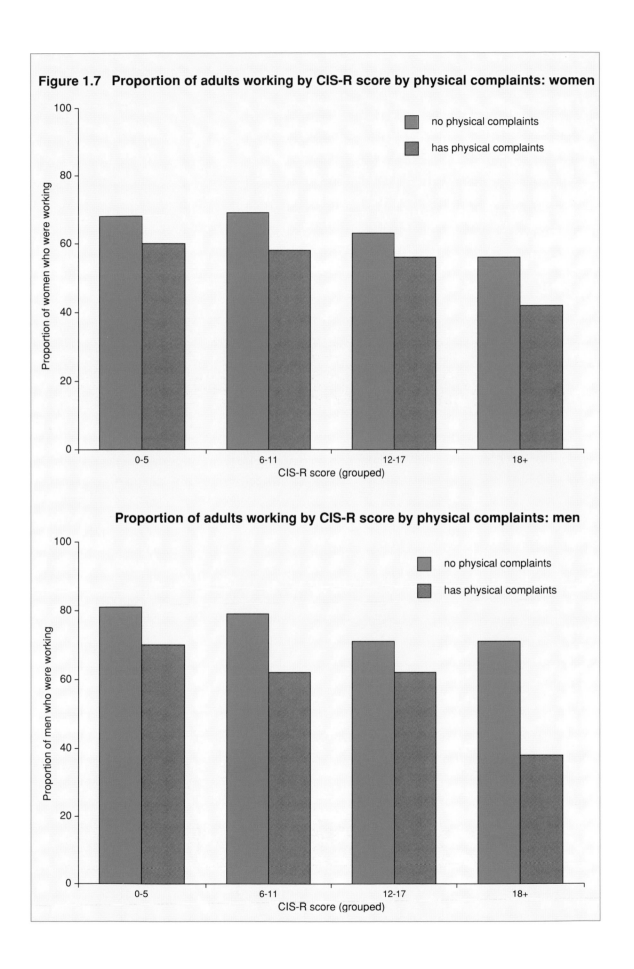

Figure 1.7 Proportion of adults working by CIS-R score by physical complaints: women

Proportion of adults working by CIS-R score by physical complaints: men

1.4 Employed people with a neurotic disorder

The mean number of days off sick in the past year varied by both number and type of neurotic disorder. Those with two or more neurotic disorders had on average 28 days a year off sick compared with 8 days per year for those with one neurotic disorder. Moreover, this finding has to be seen in the context of the proportion of each group who had been employed for at least a year: 40% of those with one neurotic disorder and 29% of those who had comorbid neuroses. Equivalent information was not collected for those without a neurotic disorder. *(Table 1.11)*

For particular disorders, there was a similar pattern for those with depressive episode or Obsessive-Compulsive Disorder: about a third had been working for at least a year and had on average about 25 days off sick in the past year. Those with phobic disorders averaged 16 days off work in the last 12 months due to illness, but only one fifth had been working for that time. *(Table 1.12)*

1.5 Unemployed people with a neurotic disorder

This section focuses on the ten percent of the sample with any neurotic disorder who were unemployed and seeking work at the time they were interviewed for the survey. *(Table 1.13)*

Among this group 70% had been unemployed for a year or more, that is, approximately 7% of all people with a neurotic disorder. About 1 in 7 of all those who were unemployed and had a neurotic disorder, regardless of how long, said that 'a mental, nervous or emotional problem' had something to do with leaving their last job.

About three quarters of this group were trying to get a full-time job. In trying to find another job, 91% had visited a Job Centre, 47% had talked to a Careers Officer, yet only 6% had spoken to a Disablement Resettlement Officer (DRO). About half of this unemployed group who had a neurotic disorder said that the way they were feeling at the moment made it more difficult for them to get a job.

1.6 Finances

Only that part of the sample who were classified as having a mental disorder were asked some basic questions about their financial circumstances: receipt of state benefits, other sources of income, and their own gross income. Comparative data from the general population were obtained from the General Household Survey or the OPCS Omnibus Survey.[3, 4]

There were significant differences between those with a neurotic disorder and the general population in the proportions receiving Income Support and Invalidity Pension, Benefit or Allowance. Compared with the general population, adults with neurosis were twice as likely to be receiving Income Support (19% compared to 10%) and four to five times more likely to be on Invalidity Benefit (9% compared to 2%). *(Table 1.14)*

In 1993, about a fifth of the general population aged 16 to 64 were in receipt of Child Benefit compared with a third of those identified in the survey as having a neurotic disorder: a ratio of 1.6 to 1. This can be explained by the higher proportion of women than men among those with neurosis: 63% compared to 38% - also a ratio of 1.6 to 1.

Taking into account the differences in economic activity between those with and without a neurotic disorder, it is not surprising to find that 47% of those with a neurotic disorder had an earned income compared with 58% of the general population. When all sources of income are added together the median weekly gross income among those with a neurotic disorder was £80-£99 compared with £140-£159 for the general population. *(Tables 1.15 and 1.16)*

References

1. Meltzer, H., Gill, B, Petticrew, M., and Hinds, K. (1995) *OPCS Surveys of Psychiatric Morbidity in Great Britain, Report* **1,** *The Prevalence of psychiatric morbidity among adults living in private households,* HMSO: London

2. Office of Population Censuses and Surveys, Series LFS no 9, (1992) *Labour Force Survey 1990 and 1991,* HMSO:London

3. Foster, K., Jackson, B., Thomas, M., Hunter, P. and Bennett, N. (1995) *General Household Survey 1993*, HMSO: London

4. Data obtained from the OPCS Omnibus Survey in 1993

Table 1.1   Economic activity of women and men by CIS-R score (grouped)

Economic activity	CIS-R score (grouped)						All
	0-5	6-11	12-17	18+	0-11	12+	
	%	%	%	%	%	%	%
Women							
Working	66	65	61	48	65	54	63
Looking for work	3	4	7	10	4	8	4
Intending to look, temporarily sick	0	1	1	3	0	2	1
Permanently unable to work	1	3	6	11	2	9	3
Retired	6	5	3	2	6	2	5
Full time education	3	4	2	4	3	3	3
Keeping house	20	18	19	22	19	20	19
Other	1	1	1	1	1	1	1
Base	*2917*	*1116*	*437*	*437*	*4034*	*874*	*4908*
Men							
Working	78	72	66	51	77	59	75
Looking for work	10	9	16	15	10	16	10
Intending to look, temporarily sick	0	2	3	3	0	3	1
Permanently unable to work	2	8	8	24	4	16	5
Retired	4	2	2	1	3	1	3
Full time education	4	5	2	6	4	4	4
Keeping house	1	2	2	0	1	1	1
Other	1	0	0	0	1	0	1
Base	*3539*	*773*	*265*	*256*	*4312*	*521*	*4833*

Table 1.2   Economic activity of women and men by CIS-R score (grouped) and age

Economic activity	CIS-R score (grouped)						All
	0-5	6-11	12-17	18+	0-11	12+	
	%	%	%	%	%	%	%
Women aged 16-39							
Working	67	66	62	48	67	54	65
Looking for work	4	5	11	12	4	12	6
Intending to look, temporarily sick	0	1	1	3	0	2	1
Permanently unable to work	1	1	2	6	1	4	1
Retired	-	-	-	-	-	-	-
Full time education	5	6	3	7	6	5	5
Keeping house	21	20	21	22	21	22	21
Other	1	1	1	1	1	1	1
Base	*1526*	*648*	*244*	*250*	*2173*	*494*	*2667*
Women aged 40-64							
Working	63	63	60	48	63	54	62
Looking for work	3	3	2	6	3	4	3
Intending to look, temporarily sick	0	0	0	3	1	2	0
Permanently unable to work	2	5	12	18	3	15	5
Retired	12	12	6	5	12	6	11
Full time education	0	1	1	0	0	0	0
Keeping house	18	14	17	20	17	19	17
Other	1	1	1	0	1	1	1
Base	*1392*	*469*	*193*	*188*	*1860*	*380*	*2241*

Table 1.2   Economic activity of women and men by CIS-R score (grouped) and age - *continued*

Economic activity	CIS-R score (grouped)						All
	0-5	6-11	12-17	18+	0-11	12+	
	%	%	%	%	%	%	%
Men aged 16-39							
Working	78	76	72	63	78	68	77
Looking for work	12	11	20	19	12	19	13
Intending to look, temporarily sick	1	1	2	3	1	2	1
Permanently unable to work	0	1	1	4	1	3	1
Retired	0	-	-	-	0	-	0
Full time education	7	9	4	11	7	7	7
Keeping house	1	2	2	-	1	1	1
Other	1	0	0	-	1	0	1
Base	*1947*	*441*	*152*	*130*	*2387*	*281*	*2669*
Men aged 40-64							
Working	77	68	60	38	75	48	72
Looking for work	7	7	11	11	7	11	7
Intending to look, temporarily sick	1	2	5	3	1	4	1
Permanently unable to work	5	17	18	45	7	32	10
Retired	8	4	4	1	8	3	7
Full time education	0	-	-	-	0	-	0
Keeping house	1	1	3	0	1	1	1
Other	1	1	-	1	1	0	1
Base	*1592*	*332*	*113*	*127*	*1924*	*240*	*2164*

Table 1.3 Economic activity of women and men by CIS-R score (grouped) and marital status

Economic activity	CIS-R score (grouped)						All
	0-5	6-11	12-17	18+	0-11	12+	
	%	%	%	%	%	%	%
Women: married or cohabiting							
Working	67	67	64	54	67	59	66
Looking for work	3	3	5	7	3	6	3
Intending to look, temporarily sick	0	0	1	3	0	2	1
Permanently unable to work	1	3	6	9	2	7	2
Retired	6	6	2	2	6	2	6
Full time education	0	1	1	0	1	1	1
Keeping house	22	19	20	24	21	22	21
Other	1	1	1	1	1	1	1
Base	*2012*	*731*	*286*	*247*	*2743*	*533*	*3276*
Women: single, widowed divorced or separated							
Working	63	61	55	40	62	46	59
Looking for work	5	6	11	13	5	12	7
Intending to look, temporarily sick	0	1	-	4	1	2	1
Permanently unable to work	2	3	7	14	2	11	4
Retired	5	4	4	2	5	3	4
Full time education	8	9	5	9	9	7	8
Keeping house	14	14	18	18	14	18	15
Other	2	1	1	1	2	1	2
Base	*892*	*380*	*150*	*191*	*1273*	*341*	*1613*

Table excludes 27 men & 18 women for whom there was no information on marital status

Table 1.3   Economic activity of women and men by CIS-R score (grouped) and marital status
- continued

Economic activity	CIS-R score (grouped)						All
	0-5	6-11	12-17	18+	0-11	12+	
	%	%	%	%	%	%	%
Men: married or cohabiting							
Working	82	78	75	56	82	64	80
Looking for work	7	6	10	12	7	11	7
Intending to look, temporarily sick	1	2	1	3	1	2	1
Permanently unable to work	3	10	8	28	4	19	6
Retired	5	2	2	1	4	2	4
Full time education	1	1	2	1	1	1	1
Keeping house	1	2	2	-	1	1	1
Other	1	0	-	-	1	-	1
Base	*2355*	*501*	*150*	*175*	*2856*	*325*	*3180*
Men: single, widowed divorced or separated							
Working	68	62	55	42	67	50	65
Looking for work	15	16	25	19	15	23	16
Intending to look, temporarily sick	1	1	6	4	1	5	1
Permanently unable to work	2	5	8	16	2	11	3
Retired	?	1	1	-	2	1	2
Full time education	10	13	2	17	11	8	10
Keeping house	1	2	1	1	1	1	1
Other	2	0	1	1	2	1	1
Base	*1165*	*268*	*113*	*80*	*1433*	*193*	*1626*

Table excludes 27 men & 18 women for whom there was no information on marital status

Table 1.4   Economic activity of women and men by CIS-R score (grouped) and qualifications

Economic activity	CIS-R score (grouped)						All
	0-5	6-11	12-17	18+	0-11	12+	
	%	%	%	%	%	%	%
Women with qualifications							
Working	72	71	69	55	71	62	72
Looking for work	3	3	7	10	3	8	4
Intending to look, temporarily sick	0	1	1	4	0	2	1
Permanently unable to work	1	2	2	5	1	4	1
Retired	4	3	1	1	4	1	3
Full time education	3	5	3	6	4	4	4
Keeping house	16	15	17	18	16	17	16
Other	1	1	0	1	1	1	1
Base	*2023*	*795*	*291*	*263*	*2818*	*555*	*3372*
Women without qualifications							
Working	52	51	45	38	52	41	50
Looking for work	4	6	7	9	5	8	5
Intending to look, temporarily sick	0	1	1	2	1	1	1
Permanently unable to work	3	6	14	20	4	17	7
Retired	11	11	6	4	11	5	10
Full time education	2	0	2	0	1	1	1
Keeping house	27	24	24	28	26	26	26
Other	1	1	1	-	1	1	1
Base	*891*	*319*	*146*	*174*	*1212*	*320*	*1530*

Table excludes 2 men & 5 women for whom there was no information on qualifications

Table 1.4   Economic activity of women and men by CIS-R score (grouped) and qualifications
            - continued

Economic activity	CIS-R score grouped						All
	0-5	6-11	12-17	18+	0-11	12+	
	%	%	%	%	%	%	%
Men with qualifications							
Working	81	80	72	63	81	68	79
Looking for work	9	6	14	14	8	14	9
Intending to look, temporarily sick	0	1	3	2	1	2	1
Permanently unable to work	1	4	5	14	2	9	2
Retired	3	2	1	-	3	1	3
Full time education	4	6	3	6	4	4	4
Keeping house	1	1	2	0	1	1	1
Other	1	0	-	-	1	-	1
Base	*2693*	*587*	*205*	*171*	*3280*	*375*	*3656*
Men without qualifications							
Working	66	49	46	26	63	34	60
Looking for work	14	18	24	16	14	20	15
Intending to look, temporarily sick	2	3	4	6	2	5	2
Permanently unable to work	7	20	18	46	10	34	12
Retired	5	2	3	2	5	2	4
Full time education	3	2	-	4	3	2	3
Keeping house	2	4	3	-	2	1	2
Other	2	1	1	1	1	1	1
Base	*844*	*186*	*60*	*86*	*1030*	*146*	*1175*

Table 1.5   Economic activity of women and men by CIS-R score (grouped) and non-manual or manual occupation

Economic activity	CIS-R score grouped						All
	0-5	6-11	12-17	18+	0-11	12+	
	%	%	%	%	%	%	%
Women in non-manual occupations							
Working	70	71	69	58	70	63	69
Looking for work	3	4	7	10	3	8	4
Intending to look, temporarily sick	0	0	-	2	0	1	1
Permanently unable to work	1	2	4	7	1	5	2
Retired	6	5	2	1	6	2	5
Full time education	2	3	1	3	2	2	2
Keeping house	17	14	17	18	17	18	17
Other	1	1	1	1	1	0	1
Base	*1522*	*564*	*204*	*189*	*2086*	*393*	*2479*
Women in manual occupations							
Working	64	61	55	42	63	48	60
Looking for work	4	4	7	9	4	8	5
Intending to look, temporarily sick	0	1	2	3	0	2	1
Permanently unable to work	2	5	9	14	3	1	4
Retired	6	5	4	3	6	3	5
Full time education	2	2	2	4	2	3	2
Keeping house	22	21	22	25	22	23	22
Other	1	1	1	1	1	0	1
Base	*1307*	*514*	*222*	*232*	*1821*	*454*	*2275*

Table excludes 170 men (48 in Armed forces, 122 with insufficient information on Social Class) and 154 women (52 in Armed forces and 102 with insufficient information on Social Class)

Table 1.5 Economic activity of women and men by CIS-R score (grouped) and non-manual or manual occupation - *continued*

Economic activity	CIS-R score (grouped)						All
	0-5	6-11	12-17	18+	0-11	12+	
	%	%	%	%	%	%	%
Men in non-manual occupations							
Working	84	82	78	66	84	73	82
Looking for work	5	7	10	11	6	11	6
Intending to look, temporarily sick	0	0	2	3	0	2	0
Permanently unable to work	2	4	5	20	2	11	3
Retired	5	2	2	-	4	1	4
Full time education	2	4	2	-	2	1	2
Keeping house	1	1	1	1	1	1	1
Other	1	0	-	-	1	-	1
Base	*1584*	*370*	*132*	*107*	*1954*	*239*	*2193*
Men in manual occupations							
Working	75	67	55	42	73	48	70
Looking for work	13	12	22	17	13	20	14
Intending to look, temporarily sick	1	3	4	4	1	4	2
Permanently unable to work	3	13	12	30	5	21	7
Retired	3	1	2	1	2	1	2
Full time education	3	1	3	5	3	4	3
Keeping house	1	2	3	-	2	1	2
Other	1	0	0	1	1	1	1
Base	*1832*	*371*	*130*	*138*	*2202*	*268*	*2471*

Table excludes 170 men (48 in Armed forces, 122 with insufficient information on Social Class) and 154 women (52 in Armed forces and 102 with insufficient information on Social Class)

Table 1.6 Economic activity of women and men by CIS-R score (grouped) and physical complaint

Economic activity	CIS-R score grouped						All
	0-5	6-11	12-17	18+	0-11	12+	
	%	%	%	%	%	%	%
Women: without physical complaint							
Working	68	69	63	56	68	61	67
Looking for work	4	4	8	10	4	9	4
Intending to look, temporarily sick	0	0	-	4	0	2	0
Permanently unable to work	0	1	1	2	0	2	1
Retired	4	3	2	1	4	1	4
Full time education	2	4	2	6	3	4	3
Keeping house	20	19	21	21	20	21	20
Other	1	1	1	-	1	0	1
Base	*2176*	*718*	*214*	*190*	*2894*	*404*	*3298*
Women: with physical complaint							
Working	60	58	56	42	59	49	58
Looking for work	3	4	6	9	3	8	4
Intending to look, temporarily sick	1	1	2	3	1	2	1
Permanently unable to work	4	8	12	18	6	15	8
Retired	11	9	4	3	10	4	8
Full time education	2	3	2	2	3	2	2
Keeping house	19	15	18	22	18	20	18
Other	1	2	1	1	1	1	1
Base	*742*	*398*	*223*	*247*	*1140*	*471*	*1610*

Table 1.6 Economic activity of women and men by CIS-R score (grouped) and physical complaint
     - continued

Economic activity	CIS-R score grouped						All
	0-5	6-11	12-17	18+	0-11	12+	
	%	%	%	%	%	%	%
Men: without physical complaint							
Working	81	79	71	71	80	71	80
Looking for work	10	9	19	16	10	18	10
Intending to look, temporarily sick	0	1	3	1	0	2	0
Permanently unable to work	0	3	1	4	1	2	1
Retired	3	1	-	1	2	0	2
Full time education	4	5	3	6	4	5	4
Keeping house	1	2	2	1	1	2	1
Other	1	0	-	1	1	0	1
Base	*2548*	*465*	*126*	*100*	*3013*	*225*	*3238*
Men: with physical complaint							
Working	70	62	62	38	68	49	64
Looking for work	9	9	14	14	9	14	10
Intending to look, temporarily sick	2	3	3	5	2	4	2
Permanently unable to work	8	15	14	37	10	26	13
Retired	6	3	3	1	6	2	5
Full time education	2	5	1	5	3	3	3
Keeping house	1	1	2	-	1	1	1
Other	1	0	0	0	1	0	1
Base	*991*	*309*	*139*	*57*	*1299*	*296*	*1595*

Table 1.7 Significant odds ratios associated with the likelihood of not working (compared with working)

Factor		Adjusted OR Intervals	95% Confidence
CIS-R score	Below threshold	1.00	....
	At or above threshold	1.52***	(1.34 - 1.74)
Physical illness	Absent	1.00	....
	Present	1.56***	(1.41 - 1.73)
Sex	Men	1.00	....
	Women	1.66***	(1.50 -1.84)
Age	16-24	1.00	....
	25-34	0.56***	(0.47 - 0.67)
	35-44	0.44***	(0.37 - 0.54)
	45-54	0.49***	(0.41 - 0.60)
	55-64	2.39***	(1.96 - 2.92)
Ethnicity	White/European	1.00	....
	West Indian/African	1.08	(0.76 - 1.54)
	Asian/Oriental	2.23***	(1.68 - 2.99)
	Other	2.02***	(1.41 - 1.73)
Family Type	Couple: no child(ren)	1.00	....
	Couple: 1+ child(ren)	1.47***	(1.29 - 1.70)
	Lone parent + child	2.57***	(2.11 - 3.12)
	One person only	1.40**	(1.21 - 1.63)
	Adult with parents	1.49**	(1.16 - 1.90)
	Adult with one parent	1.40***	(1.05 - 1.88)
Qualifications	A Level or higher	1.00	....
	GCSE/O Level	1.31***	(1.14 - 1.50)
	Other	1.52***	(1.28 - 1.80)
	None	2.17***	(1.89 - 2.49)
Tenure	Owner/Occupier	1.00	....
	Renter	2.51***	(2.23 - 2.82)
Occupation type	Non-manual	1.00	....
	Manual	1.23***	(1.11 - 1.37)
Accommodation	Detached	1.00	....
	Semi-detached	0.76***	(0.66 - 0.88)
	Terraced	0.88	(0.76 - 1.02)
	Flat/Maisonette	0.86	(0.73 - 1.03)

* p< 0.05   ** p< 0.01   ***p<0.001

Table 1.8 Proportions of adults who are permanently unable to work and their characteristics by CIS-R score

Characteristics*	CIS-R score: 12+	CIS-R score: 0-11
	Proportion permanently unable to work owing to long-term sickness or disability	
Men, aged 40-64, in manual occupations	42% (122)	10% (966)
Men, aged 40-64, in non-manual occupations	22% (117)	4% (942)
Women, aged 40-64, in manual occupations	19% (217)	4% (851)
Women, aged 40-64, in non-manual occupations	10% (158)	2% (990)
Women, aged 16-39, in manual occupations	4% (237)	1% (970)
Men, aged 16-39, in manual occupations	3% (147)	1% (1237)
Women, aged 16-39, in non-manual occupations	2% (235)	1% (1096)
Men, aged 16-39 in non-manual occupations	2% (122)	0% (1012)

* Classification of occupation was based on last job

Bases in brackets

Table 1.9 Economic activity by number of disorders by sex

Economic activity	No neurotic disorder	One neurotic disorder	Two or more neurotic disorders	All
	%	%	%	%
Women				
Working	65	58	33	63
Looking for work	4	8	10	4
Intending to look, temporarily sick	0	2	5	1
Permanently unable to work	2	7	20	3
Retired	6	3	1	5
Full time education	3	3	5	3
Keeping house	19	19	26	19
Other	1	1	1	1
Base	*3948*	*830*	*130*	*4908*
Men				
Working	77	61	46	75
Looking for work	10	16	15	10
Intending to look, temporarily sick	1	3	3	1
Permanently unable to work	3	14	30	5
Retired	3	1	-	3
Full time education	4	4	3	4
Keeping house	1	1	1	1
Other	1	0	1	1
Base	*4236*	*519*	*79*	*4833*

Table 1.10 Economic activity of adults with neurotic disorders by sex

Economic activity	Mixed anxiety and depressive disorder	GAD	Depressive episode	Phobias	OCD	Panic	Any neurotic disorder	No neurotic disorder	All
	%	%	%	%	%	%	%	%	%
Women									
Working	60	46	41	30	47	58	54	66	63
Looking for work	9	8	7	9	8	5	8	4	4
Intending to look, temporarily sick	1	2	6	16	4	-	2	0	1
Permanently unable to work	6	14	13	20	16	6	9	2	3
Retired	3	5	1	2	1	4	3	6	5
Full time education	3	4	3	11	4	1	3	3	3
Keeping house	19	22	27	22	19	27	20	19	19
Other	1	0	3	1	2	-	1	1	1
Base	*485*	*251*	*133*	*122*	*100*	*50*	*960*	*3948*	*4908*
Men									
Working	63	55	50	43	54	53	59	77	75
Looking for work	14	16	16	20	18	19	16	10	10
Intending to look, temporarily sick	3	4	4	4	2	4	3	1	1
Permanently unable to work	12	22	25	20	24	15	16	3	5
Retired	1	1	-	1	-	3	1	3	3
Full time education	5	0	3	8	3	6	4	4	4
Keeping house	1	1	1	2	-	-	1	1	1
Other	0	-	1	2	-	-	0	1	1
Base	*265*	*188*	*88*	*58*	*57*	*43*	*597*	*4236*	*4833*

25

Table 1.11 Mean number of 'days off work due to ill health' in past year by number of neurotic disorders and sex

	One neurotic disorder	Two or more neurotic disorders	Any neurotic disorder
Proportion employed for one year or more	40% *(1349)*	29% *(209)*	38% *(1557)*
Mean number of days off work in past year			
All	8 *(538)*	28 *(60)*	10 *(599)*
Women	8 *(333)*	22 *(33)*	9 *(366)*
Men	9 *(206)*	35 *(27)*	12 *(233)*

Bases in brackets

Table 1.12 Mean number of 'days off work due to ill health' in past year by type of disorder

	Mixed anxiety and depressive disorder	Generalised Anxiety Disorder	Depressive episode	Phobias	Obsessive-Compulsive Disorder	Panic	Any neurotic disorder
Proportion employed for one year or more	47%	30%	32%	20%	31%	34%	38%
Base = number with disorder	750	439	220	180	157	93	1557
Mean number of days off work in past year	7	15	25	16	23	10	10
Base = number of people employed for one year or more	351	130	71	36	48	32	599

Table 1.13 Behaviour and attitudes of those with a neurotic disorder who were unemployed and seeking work

Factors relating to last job

Time since last worked	%
Less than 1 year	30
1 < 2 years	26
2 < 3 years	14
3 < 4 years	9
4 < 5 years	7
5 or more years	14

Whether a mental, nervous or emotional problem had anything to do with leaving last job	
Yes	14
No	86

Factors related to seeking work

Has visited a Job Centre	%
Yes	91
No	9

Has talked to a Careers Officer	
Yes	47
No	53

Has talked to a Disablement Resettlement Officer (DRO)	
Yes	6
No	94

Has the 'way you are feeling' made it more difficult for you to find a job ?	
Yes	46
No	54

Preference for full or part time work	
Full time	78
Part time	22

Base (unemployed and seeking work)	*153*

Table 1.14 Receipt of State Benefits

State benefit	Percentage of adults with neurotic disorder getting each type of State Benefit	Percentage of adults (from GHS) getting each type of State Benefit*
Child Benefit	32	22
Income Support	19	10
Invalidity pension, benefit or allowance	9	2
Sickness Benefit	3	0
Unemployment Benefit	3	2
Family Credit	2	1
Old Age pension	2	3
Mobility Allowance	2	..
Disability Living Allowance	2	2
Attendance Allowance	1	-
Industrial Disablement Allowance	1	0
Widow's pension or War Widow's pension	1	0
Severe Disablement Allowance	1	0
Invalid Care Allowance	1	1
Widowed Mother's Allowance	0	0
War Disablement pension	0	0
Disability Working Allowance	0	0
Base	*1557*	*13744*

.. Data not available

* General Household Survey 1993

Table 1.15   Summary of sources of income

Source of Income	Percentage of adults with neurotic disorder who have each source of income	Percentage of all adults (from GHS) who have each source of income*
Earned income or salary	47	58
Income from self- employment	8	8
Pension from a former employer	5	5
Interest from savings, building society, investment dividends from shares etc	26	..
Any other type of regular allowance from outside the household (eg alimony, annuity, educational grant etc)	5	6
Base	*1557*	*13744*

.. Data unavailable

* Data from the 1993 General Household Survey

Table 1.16   Personal Gross Income

Yearly income	Weekly income	% of those with a neurotic disorder		% of the whole population (from the 1993 Omnibus Survey)	
Less than £1000	Less than £20	12		7	
£1000 to £1999	£20 - £39	8		7	
£2000 to £2999	£40 - £ 59	9	51	9	39
£3000 to £3999	£60 - £79	13		9	
£4000 to £4999	£80 - £99	9		7	
£5000 to £5999	£100 - £119	7		6	
£6000 to £6999	£120 - £139	5		5	
£7000 to £7999	£140 - £159	4	23	5	24
£8000 to £8999	£160 - £179	4		4	
£9000 to £9999	£180 - £199	3		4	
£10000 to £10999	£200 - £219	3		4	
£11000 to £11999	£220 - £239	3		3	
£12000 to £12999	£240 - £259	2	12	3	16
£13000 to £13999	£260 - £ 279	1		2	
£14000 to £14999	£280 - £299	3		3	
£15000 to £17499	£300 - £349	3		5	
£17500 to £19999	£350 - £399	3		4	
£20000 to £24999	£400 - £499	3	13	5	20
£25000 to £29999	£500 - £599	2		2	
£30000 or more	£600 or more	2		4	
Median weekly income		£80 - £99		£140 - £159	
Base		*1557*		*18,760*	

*Data from the 1993 OPCS Omnibus Survey

2 Activities of daily living (ADL)

2.1 Introduction

All 10,108 adults interviewed in the survey were asked about any difficulty they had with particular activities of daily living. The selection of activities was influenced by the topics covered in the MRC Needs for Care Assessment[1], and the OPCS Surveys of Disability[2]. The seven areas of functioning covered by the survey were:

- **Personal care** such as dressing, bathing, washing, or using the toilet.

- **Using transport** to get out and about.

- **Medical care** such as taking medicines or pills, having injections or changes of dressing.

- **Household activities** such as preparing meals, shopping, laundry and housework.

- **Practical activities** such as gardening, decorating or doing household repairs.

- **Dealing with paperwork**, such as writing letters, sending cards or filling in forms.

- **Managing money** such as budgeting for food or paying bills.

If respondents said they had any difficulty with these activities, they were asked whether they needed help, and if so, who provided it. This chapter looks at all these aspects in terms of our general measure of neurotic psychopathology (the CIS-R score) and by particular neurotic disorders. In all tables, data are presented according to whether or not those interviewed had a physical illness as this has a major

influence on difficulties with ADL[3].

2.2 ADL and the overall CIS-R score

Fifteen percent of all adults reported having a difficulty with at least one activity of daily living. Those on or above the threshold score of 12 on the CIS-R were nearly three times more likely to have any ADL difficulty than those with subthreshold scores (33% compared with 12%). There is practically a linear progression in the proportions of adults with any ADL difficulty in the four CIS-R groups: from 10% among the lowest scorers to 40% of those with scores of 18 or more.*(Table 2.1 & Figure 2.1)*

As expected, physical illness has a major effect on the ability to carry out the whole range of tasks irrespective of the presence of a neurotic health problem. Adults with a physical disorder were three times more likely than those without a physical illness to have ADL difficulties: 28% compared with 9%. A neurotic health problem with a physical illness adds to the level of difficulty. Among those without a physical or mental health problem (CIS-R score below 12), 8% had difficulty with at least one ADL, whereas among those with both types of health problem, the equivalent proportion was 45%, almost a six-fold increase. Having difficulty with any activity is a general measure of ADL performance. Table 2.1 also shows the number of tasks with which respondents had difficulty. Focusing on proportions of adults with two or more ADL difficulties, 2% of the group without any physical or health problem were in this situation compared with 28% of those with both types of problem. The most severely affected group were those who had a physical illness and a score of 18 or more on the CIS-R; just over half (52%) had at least one ADL difficulty and

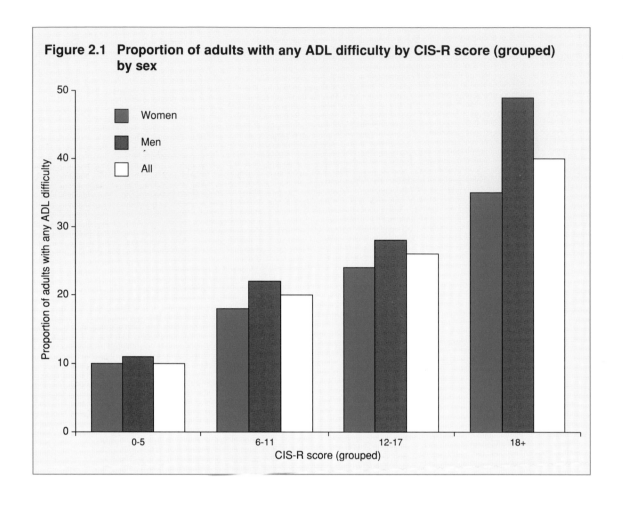

Figure 2.1 Proportion of adults with any ADL difficulty by CIS-R score (grouped) by sex

37% were limited in performing two or more tasks. *(Table 2.1)*

In Table 2.2, the seven activities of daily living are listed in descending order of the proportions of adults who had difficulties carrying out the tasks across the whole population. The most problematic activities were practical tasks - gardening, decorating or doing household repairs whereas people had the least difficulty in managing their medicinal regimes or other forms of medical care.

Looking at the whole sample, the trend of increasing proportions of people having difficulty with increasing CIS-R scores was evident for all activities of daily living.

Physical illness had its most noticeable effect on activities which required physical exertion -

practical activities, household activities and use of transport. For instance, among those with a score of 12+ on the CIS-R and who had a physical health problem, 18% had difficulty getting out and about using transport. This is in contrast to the 6% who had a physical illness and a subthreshold CIS-R score, and the 3% with a neurotic health problem and no physical health problem. The equivalent percentages for practical activities were 30%, 13% and 6%. The activities which did not show this pattern were managing money and to a lesser extent dealing with paperwork. Not surprisingly, the proportions of people in each of the four CIS-R groups with difficulty managing money hardly varied by the existence or absence of a physical illness: 12% of those with a CIS-R score of 18+ had difficulty managing money regardless of whether they had any physical complaint. *(Table 2.2)*

30

2.3 ADL and the neurotic disorders

In Table 2.3, another dimension, the number of neurotic disorders, is added into the analysis. Variability in proportions of people with ADL difficulties was related to all three factors: the presence of a physical disorder, the existence of a neurotic disorder and the extent of comorbid neurotic disorders.

Among adults reporting no physical health problem, 35% of those with two neurotic disorders had at least one ADL difficulty, practically twice the proportion of those with one neurotic disorder (19%), and over four times the proportion without a neurotic disorder (8%). A similar relationship was found for those with a physical illness; 69% of the group with 2 neurotic disorders had difficulty with at least one ADL activity compared with 40% of those with one neurotic disorder and 22% of adults who just had a physical disorder. *(Table 2.3)*

For almost all the activities of daily living, those with comorbid neurotic disorders were two to three times more likely to experience some difficulty than the group with one neurotic disorder.

2.4 The association between neurotic disorders and ADL

In order to examine the independent association of neurotic disorders with particular activities of daily living, logistic regression was used. The independent variables, the ADL, were dichotomised into whether or not people had difficulty with each task. In terms of the explanatory factors, it has already been clearly demonstrated that factors such as physical illness and comorbidity among the neurotic disorders are of great importance. Other factors entered in the model were four socio-demographic characteristics: sex, age, family type, and educational attainment. Sex was chosen because certain activities of daily living are traditionally carried out more by one sex than

another. Similarly, family type can have an effect because certain tasks may be delegated to other family members. Age is an important factor as it is highly correlated with physical disability and educational achievement was put in the model as a broad measure of competence.

Each of the six factors entered in the model show significant odds ratios for some activity of daily living. Our interest is in the independent relationship of having a neurotic disorder and the performance of these tasks, ie controlling for physical illness, age, sex etc. The large increase in the odds ratios of having difficulty with any ADL for the groups with neurotic disorders compared with the non-case reference group is striking. For individuals with one neurotic disorder the increase in odds ranges from OR=2.26 (dealing with paperwork) to OR=4.34 (personal care). For those with comorbid neurotic disorders, the range extended from OR=4.87 (dealing with paperwork) to OR=10.10 (use of transport). *(Table 2.4)*

2.5 ADL and specific neurotic disorders

The relationship between number of disorders and the ADL difficulties may explain why people with phobia, depressive episode and OCD have the highest proportions with any ADL difficulty, 55%, 45% and 42% as these three groups have the greatest extent of neurotic comorbidity. *(Table 2.5)*

The relationship between specific neurotic disorders and particular ADL difficulties is most clearly seen for those without a physical illness, the top sections of Tables 2.5 and 2.6 because the confounding effect of the physical illness has been removed. For this group, difficulties in activities of daily living may reflect the symptoms of the disorders.

Forty five percent of people with a phobia (without a longstanding physical illness) had difficulty with at least one activity of daily living. The next most affected groups were those with a depressive episode or OCD, where just over a quarter had some difficulty. Among those with a depressive disorder, 12% had problems with three or more tasks, the highest proportion on this measure across all groups. *(Table 2.5)*

Looking at specific activities, again among those without a physical disorder, between 10 and 20 percent of adults with GAD, depressive episode, phobias or OCD experienced difficulty with managing money or with dealing with paperwork. Among the sample with a physical and neurotic disorder, the two activities affecting the largest proportion were practical activities (30%) and household activities (22%).
(Table 2.6)

2.6   ADL and the need for help

Over two thirds of people with a neurotic disorder who had difficulty with practical activities, household activities, dealing with paperwork, using transport or personal care said they needed help. Managing money was different in that just half mentioned help was

required with this task. Nearly, all those who needed help got assistance. These findings were evident for people with or without a physical disorder as well as a neurotic disorder. *(Table 2.7)*

The vast majority of help was provided by a close relative. Friends made a helpful contribution to those who had difficulties getting out and about using transport. Just over a quarter of people with such difficulties had help from friends. *(Table 2.8)*

References

1. Brewin, C.R. and Wing, J.K., (1989) *MRC Needs for Care assessment*, MRC Social Psychiatry Unit, Institute of Psychiatry, London.

2. Martin, J., Meltzer, H., and Elliot, D., (1988) *The OPCS Surveys of Disability in Great Britain, Report 1, The prevalence of disability among adults*, HMSO, London.

3. Martin, J., White, A., and Meltzer, H., (1989) *The OPCS Surveys of Disability in Great Britain, Report 4, Disabled Adults: Services, Transport and Employment*, HMSO, London.

Table 2.1   Number of ADL difficulties by CIS-R score by physical complaint

	CIS-R score (grouped)						All
	0-5	6-11	12-17	18+	0-11	12+	
	%	%	%	%	%	%	%
Without physical complaint							
0	93	85	85	76	92	81	91
1	6	10	8	14	6	11	7
2	1	3	4	6	1	5	2
3	0	2	2	3	1	2	1
4	0	-	1	1	0	1	0
5+	0	0	-	1	0	0	0
Percentage with any ADL difficulty	**7**	**15**	**15**	**24**	**8**	**19**	**9**
Base	*4724*	*1183*	*340*	*289*	*5906*	*629*	*6535*
With physical complaint							
0	80	72	64	48	78	55	72
1	12	14	17	15	13	16	14
2	4	7	7	10	5	8	6
3	2	3	6	10	2	8	4
4	1	2	3	9	2	6	3
5+	1	2	4	8	1	6	2
Percentage with any ADL difficulty	**20**	**28**	**36**	**52**	**22**	**45**	**28**
Base	*1732*	*707*	*362*	*404*	*2439*	*767*	*3206*
All adults							
0	90	80	74	60	88	67	85
1	7	12	13	15	8	14	9
2	2	5	6	8	2	7	3
3	1	2	4	7	1	6	2
4	0	1	2	6	1	4	1
5+	0	1	2	5	0	3	1
Percentage with any ADL difficulty	**10**	**20**	**26**	**40**	**12**	**33**	**15**
Base	*6456*	*1890*	*702*	*694*	*8346*	*1396*	*9741*

Table 2.2 Type of ADL difficulties by CIS-R score by physical complaint

	CIS-R score (grouped)						All
	0-5	6-11	12-17	18+	0-11	12+	
Percentage who had difficulty with each task							
Without physical complaint							
Practical activities	1	4	4	7	2	6	2
Dealing with paperwork	4	6	5	10	4	8	4
Household activities	1	2	3	4	1	3	1
Using transport	1	2	1	4	1	3	1
Managing money	2	6	8	12	3	10	4
Personal care	0	1	1	1	0	1	0
Medical care	0	1	0	2	1	1	1
Base	*4724*	*1183*	*340*	*289*	*5906*	*629*	*6535*
With a physical complaint							
Practical activities	11	18	24	36	13	30	17
Dealing with paperwork	7	8	12	21	7	17	10
Household activities	5	9	16	27	6	22	10
Using transport	5	8	10	26	6	18	9
Managing money	2	5	9	12	3	11	5
Personal care	3	5	7	18	4	13	6
Medical care	1	1	2	3	1	2	1
Base	*1732*	*707*	*362*	*404*	*2439*	*767*	*3206*
All adults							
Practical activities	4	9	14	24	5	18	7
Dealing with paperwork	4	7	9	17	5	13	6
Household activities	2	5	10	17	3	13	4
Using transport	2	4	6	17	2	11	4
Managing money	2	6	9	12	3	10	4
Personal care	1	2	4	11	1	8	2
Medical care	0	1	1	2	1	2	1
Base	*6456*	*1890*	*702*	*694*	*8346*	*1396*	*9741*

Table 2.3 Number and type of ADL difficulties by number of neurotic disorders by physical complaint

		No physical complaint			Has physical complaint		
		No neurotic disorder	1 neurotic disorder	2+ neurotic disorders	No neurotic disorder	1 neurotic disorder	2+ neurotic disorders
		%	%	%	%	%	%
No. of ADL difficulties							
	0	92	81	66	78	60	31
	1	6	12	14	13	14	26
	2	1	5	10	5	8	12
	3	1	2	7	2	7	14
	4	0	0	2	2	5	11
	5+	0	0	1	1	6	6
Percentage with any difficulty		**8**	**19**	**35**	**22**	**40**	**69**
Percentage with each type of difficulty							
Practical activities		2	6	10	13	28	38
Dealing with paperwork		4	7	17	7	15	27
Household activities		1	3	10	6	20	30
Use of transport		1	3	9	6	16	33
Managing money		3	8	18	3	10	16
Personal care		0	2	2	4	11	22
Medical care		1	1	3	1	2	2
Base		*5751*	*697*	*87*	*2433*	*651*	*121*

Table 2.4   Odds ratios of the correlates of ADL difficulties

		Practical activities	Dealing with paperwork	Household activities
		OR (95%CI)	OR (95%CI)	OR (95%CI)
Neurotic Disorders	0	1.00	1.00	1.00 ....
	1	3.31*** (2.73-4.00)	2.26*** (1.83-2.79)	3.71*** (2.94-4.68)
	2+	5.08*** (3.54-7.29)	4.87*** (3.39-7.02)	7.28***(4.95-10.72)
Physical Disorder	Absent	1.00	1.00	1.00 . ...
	Present	6.35*** (5.22-7.73)	1.68*** (1.40-2.02)	6.27*** (4.84-8.13)
Age	16-24	1.00	1.00	1.00 ....
	25-34	1.29 (0.84-2.01)	0.83 (0.59-1.18)	1.60* (1.02-2.52)
	35-44	1.98** (1.28-3.05)	0.79 (0.55-1.13)	1.78* (1.15-2.78)
	45-54	2.88*** (1.89-4.40)	0.74 (0.52-1.07)	2.38*** (1.54-3.67)
	55-64	4.64*** (3.05-7.08)	1.13 (0.79-1.63)	3.17*** (2.05-4.89)
Sex	Men	-	1.00	1.00 ....
	Women	-	0.50*** (0.41-0.60)	1.84*** (1.47-2.31)
Family unit type	Couple, no child(ren	1.00	1.00	-
	Couple & child(ren)	0.82 (0.66-1.01)	1.27* (1.01-1.62)	-
	Lone parent & child(ren)	1.28 (0.91-1.81)	1.40 (0.94-2.08)	-
	One person only	1.02 (0.79-1.32)	1.55** (1.18-2.03)	-
	Adult with parents	0.34** (0.19-0.74)	0.71 (0.45-1.14)	-
	Adult with one parent	1.10 (0.60-2.02)	1.16 (0.68-1.99)	-
Qualifications	Any	-	1.00	1.00 ....
	None	-	2.22*** (2.76-4.01)	1.28* (1.02-1.61)

* p<0.05;   ** p<0.01;   *** p<0.001

Table 2.4   Odds ratios of the correlates of ADL difficulties - *continued*

		Using transport OR (95%CI)	Managing money OR (95%CI)	Personal care OR (95%CI)
Neurotic Disorders	0	1.00	1.00	1.00 ....
	1	3.72*** (2.89-4.80)	2.92*** (2.30-3.72)	4.34*** (3.18-5.94)
	2+	10.10*** (6.83-14.95.)	6.07*** (4.05-9.10)	9.27***(5.76-14.93)
Physical Disorder	Absent	1.00	1.00	1.00 . ...
	Present	6.45*** (4.82-8.64)	1.27*** (1.01-1.58)	8.76*** (5.75-13.34)
Age	16-24	1.00	1.00	1.00 ....
	25-34	1.23 (0.23-2.08)	0.78 (0.57-1.08)	0.78 (0.37-1.62)
	35-44	1.99** (1.22-2.34)	0.47*** (0.32-0.68)	1.58 (0.83-3.02)
	45-54	2.15*** (1.32-3.48)	0.31*** (0.21-0.48)	2.59** (1.41-4.78)
	55-64	3.44*** (2.14-5.53)	0.42*** (0.79-1.63)	5.22*** (2.89-9.44)
Sex	Men	-	1.00	-
	Women	-	0.58*** (0.46-0.72)	-
Family unit type	Couple, no child(ren	-	1.00	-
	Couple & child(ren)	-	1.42* (1.02-1.98)	-
	Lone parent & child(ren)	-	2.87*** (1.84-4.46)	-
	One person only	-	2.23*** (1.56-3.19)	-
	Adult with parents	-	1.48 (0.94-2.32)	-
	Adult with one parent	-	2.50*** (1.50-4.20)	-
Qualifications	Any	1.00	1.00	-
	None	1.69*** (1.32-2.15)	1.71*** (1.36-2.17)	-

* p<0.05;   ** p<0.01;   *** p<0.001

Table 2.5   Number of ADL difficulties by type of neurotic illness by whether or not has physical complaint

	Mixed anxiety and depressive disorder	Generalised Anxiety Disorder	Depression	Phobia	Obsessive Compulsive Disorder	Panic	Any neurotic disorder	No neurotic disorder	All
	%	%	%	%	%	%	%	%	%
Without a physical complaint									
0	88	72	72	55	73	86	79	92	91
1	8	16	15	20	13	8	12	6	7
2	3	7	2	16	10	-	5	1	2
3	1	4	9	7	2	4	3	1	1
4	0	1	2	1	2	-	1	0	0
5+	-	1	1	1	1	2	0	0	0
Percentage with any ADL difficulty	**12**	**28**	**28**	**45**	**27**	**14**	**21**	**8**	**9**
Base	*351*	*232*	*106*	*95*	*71*	*46*	*784*	*5751*	*6535*
With a physical complaint									
0	63	45	39	34	46	52	56	78	72
1	13	20	20	28	20	15	16	13	14
2	8	10	8	10	7	10	8	5	6
3	5	10	14	15	12	10	8	2	4
4	5	8	11	9	10	10	6	2	3
5+	5	6	9	5	5	3	6	1	2
Percentage with any ADL difficulty	**37**	**55**	**61**	**66**	**54**	**48**	**44**	**22**	**28**
Base	*399*	*207*	*115*	*85*	*86*	*47*	*773*	*2433*	*3206*
All adults									
0	75	59	55	45	58	69	68	88	85
1	11	18	18	24	17	12	14	8	9
2	6	8	5	13	8	5	7	2	3
3	3	7	12	10	8	7	5	1	2
4	3	4	6	5	6	5	3	0	1
5+	3	3	5	3	3	3	3	0	1
Percentage with any ADL difficulty	**25**	**41**	**45**	**55**	**42**	**31**	**32**	**12**	**15**
Base	*750*	*439*	*220*	*180*	*157*	*93*	*1557*	*8184*	*9741*

Table 2.6   Type of ADL difficulties by type of neurotic illness by physical complaint

	Mixed anxiety and depressive disorder	Generalised Anxiety Disorder	Depression	Phobia	Obsessive-Compulsive Disorder	Panic	Any neurotic disorder	No neurotic disorder	All
Percentage who had difficulty with each task									
Without physical complaint									
Practical activities	4	10	9	14	9	5	7	2	2
Dealing with paperwork	4	13	14	18	13	9	8	4	4
Household activities	2	5	7	10	6	4	4	1	1
Using transport	1	6	5	15	10	5	4	1	1
Managing money	7	10	16	19	11	3	9	3	4
Personal care	0	3	4	3	2	2	2	0	0
Medical care	1	1	2	2	-	2	1	1	1
Base	*351*	*232*	*106*	*95*	*71*	*46*	*784*	*5751*	*6535*
With physical complaint									
Practical activities	28	32	41	35	31	23	30	13	17
Dealing with paperwork	13	23	23	24	22	21	17	7	10
Household activities	19	25	33	31	21	23	22	6	10
Using transport	14	24	27	29	28	21	18	6	9
Managing money	7	15	19	14	11	12	10	3	5
Personal care	9	17	20	18	22	14	13	4	6
Medical care	2	2	4	-	1	6	2	1	1
Base	*399*	*207*	*115*	*85*	*86*	*47*	*773*	*2433*	*3206*
All adults									
Practical activities	16	21	26	24	21	14	18	5	7
Dealing with paperwork	9	18	19	21	18	15	12	5	6
Household activities	11	15	21	20	14	14	13	2	4
Using transport	8	14	17	22	20	13	11	2	4
Managing money	7	12	18	16	11	8	10	3	4
Personal care	5	10	12	10	12	8	7	1	2
Medical care	2	1	3	1	1	4	2	1	1
Base	*750*	*439*	*220*	*180*	*157*	*93*	*1557*	*8184*	*9741*

39

Table 2.7   Need for help by type of ADL difficulty by neurotic disorder by physical complaint

	Mixed anxiety and depressive disorder	Generalised Anxiety Disorder	Depression	Phobia	Obsessive-Compulsive Disorder	Panic	Any neurotic disorder	No neurotic disorder	All
No physical complaint	%	%	%	%	%	%	%	%	%
Practical activities									
Has difficulty									
needs help, gets help	2	7	4	11	3	4	4	1	2
needs help, gets no help	0	1	1	-	2	-	0	0	0
needs no help	1	2	3	2	3	1	2	0	1
Has no difficulty	97	90	92	87	92	95	93	98	98
Household activities									
Has difficulty									
needs help, gets help	1	4	5	8	4	2	3	1	1
needs help, gets no help	-	1	1	0	0	2	0	0	0
needs no help	1	0	0	1	2	-	1	0	0
Has no difficulty	98	95	93	90	94	96	96	99	99
Dealing with paperwork									
Has difficulty									
needs help, gets help	2	8	13	13	7	6	5	3	3
needs help, gets no help	-	1	-	-	-	-	0	0	0
needs no help	2	4	1	4	5	3	3	1	1
Has no difficulty	96	88	86	83	88	91	92	96	96
Using transport									
Has difficulty									
needs help, gets help	0	4	2	9	7	5	2	0	1
needs help, gets no help	-	-	-	-	-	-	-	-	-
needs no help	0	2	2	8	4	-	1	0	0
Has no difficulty	99	94	95	86	90	95	96	100	99
Managing money									
Has difficulty									
needs help, gets help	2	4	5	5	3	2	3	1	1
needs help, gets no help	1	1	1	-	-	-	1	0	0
needs no help	4	5	10	14	7	1	5	2	2
Has no difficulty	93	90	84	82	90	97	91	97	96
Personal care									
Has difficulty									
needs help, gets help	-	2	-	0	-	2	1	0	0
needs help, gets no help	-	-	-	-	-	-	-	-	-
needs no help	0	2	4	2	2	-	1	0	0
Has no difficulty	99	97	96	98	98	98	98	100	100
Medical care									
Has difficulty									
needs help, gets help	0	0	1	-	-	2	0	0	0
needs help, gets no help	-	-	-	-	-	-	-	-	-
needs no help	0	0	1	2	-	-	0	0	0
Has no difficulty	99	99	98	98	100	98	99	100	100
Base	*351*	*232*	*106*	*95*	*71*	*46*	*784*	*5751*	*6535*

Table 2.7   Need for help by type of ADL difficulty by neurotic disorder by physical complaint - *continued*

	Mixed anxiety and depressive disorder	Generalised Anxiety Disorder	Depression	Phobia	Obsessive Compulsive Disorder	Panic	Any neurotic disorder	No neurotic disorder	All
With physical complaint	%	%	%	%	%	%	%	%	%
Practical activities									
Has difficulty									
needs help, gets help	22	26	33	28	29	18	24	10	13
needs help, gets no help	1	1	2	3	1	-	1	0	0
needs no help	5	5	6	5	1	6	5	3	4
Has no difficulty	73	68	59	65	68	77	70	87	83
Household activities									
Has difficulty									
needs help, gets help	15	19	26	27	15	18	17	5	8
needs help, gets no help	0	1	1	2	1	1	1	0	0
needs no help	3	6	6	1	4	4	4	1	2
Has no difficulty	81	75	68	70	80	77	78	94	90
Dealing with paperwork									
Has difficulty									
needs help, gets help	10	17	17	16	20	11	12	6	7
needs help, gets no help	0	1	0	2	-	4	1	0	0
needs no help	3	5	6	7	2	6	4	2	2
Has no difficulty	87	77	77	76	78	79	83	93	91
Using transport									
Has difficulty									
needs help, gets help	9	12	12	18	21	9	11	3	5
needs help, gets no help	0	-	1	-	-	-	0	0	0
needs no help	5	12	14	11	7	11	7	3	4
Has no difficulty	86	77	73	71	72	80	82	94	91
Managing money									
Has difficulty									
needs help, gets help	4	8	10	6	6	6	5	2	3
needs help, gets no help	0	1	0	2	1	1	1	-	0
needs no help	3	6	8	4	4	5	4	1	2
Has no difficulty	93	85	81	87	90	88	90	97	95
Personal care									
Has difficulty									
needs help, gets help	6	10	15	14	15	9	8	2	4
needs help, gets no help	0	0	0	1	-	-	0	0	0
needs no help	4	7	5	4	7	5	4	1	2
Has no difficulty	91	83	80	82	78	86	87	96	94
Medical care									
Has difficulty									
needs help, gets help	1	0	1	-	0	5	1	1	1
needs help, gets no help	-	-	-	-	-	-	-	-	-
needs no help	1	1	3	-	0	1	1	0	0
Has no difficulty	98	98	96	100	99	94	98	99	99
Base	*399*	*206*	*115*	*85*	*86*	*47*	*773*	*2433*	*3206*

Table 2.7   Need for help by type of ADL difficulty by neurotic disorder by physical complaint - *continued*

	Mixed anxiety and depressive disorder	Generalised Anxiety Disorder	Depression	Phobia	Obsessive Compulsive Disorder	Panic	Any neurotic disorder	No neurotic disorder	All
All adults	%	%	%	%	%	%	%	%	%
Practical activities									
Has difficulty									
needs help, gets help	12	16	20	19	17	11	14	4	5
needs help, gets no help	0	1	2	1	2	-	1	0	0
needs no help	3	4	4	3	2	3	3	1	2
Has no difficulty	84	79	74	77	79	86	82	95	93
Household activities									
Has difficulty									
needs help, get help	8	11	16	17	10	10	10	2	3
needs help, gets no help	0	0	1	1	1	2	0	0	0
needs no help	2	4	3	1	3	2	2	1	1
Has no difficulty	89	85	80	81	86	86	88	98	96
Dealing with paperwork									
Has difficulty									
needs help, gets help	6	12	15	14	14	9	9	4	4
needs help, gets no help	0	1	0	1	-	2	0	0	0
needs no help	3	4	3	5	3	4	3	1	1
Has no difficulty	91	83	82	80	83	85	88	95	94
Using transport									
Has difficulty									
needs help, gets help	5	8	7	13	15	7	7	1	2
needs help, gets no help	0	-	1	-	-	-	0	0	0
needs no help	3	6	8	8	5	5	4	1	1
Has no difficulty	82	86	84	79	80	88	89	98	96
Managing money									
Has difficulty									
needs help, gets help	5	6	8	5	4	4	4	1	2
needs help, gets no help	1	1	1	1	0	1	1	0	0
needs no help	6	6	9	9	5	3	5	2	2
Has no difficulty	88	88	83	84	90	92	90	97	96
Personal care									
Has difficulty									
needs help, gets help	3	6	8	7	8	5	4	1	1
needs help, gets no help	0	0	-	0	-	-	0	0	0
needs no help	2	4	4	3	4	3	2	0	1
Has no difficulty	95	90	88	90	88	92	93	99	98
Medical care									
Has difficulty									
needs help, gets help	1	1	1	-	0	4	1	0	0
needs help, gets no help	-	-	-	-	-	-	-	-	-
needs no help	1	1	2	1	0	1	1	0	0
Has no difficulty	98	98	97	99	99	96	98	99	99
Base	*750*	*439*	*220*	*180*	*157*	*93*	*1557*	*8184*	*9241*

Table 2.8   Type of helper by type of difficulty

	Practical activities	Household activities	Paperwork	Using transport	Managing money	Personal care	Medical care
Percentage of those with difficulty receiving help*							
Spouse/cohabitee	54	48	49	54	51	80	[9]
Brother/sister	10	5	10	12	8	5	[2]
Son/daughter	30	31	17	34	3	20	[2]
Parent	6	10	16	12	25	6	-
Grandparent	-	-	1	-	-	-	-
Grandchild	0	0	0	1	-	2	-
Other relative	2	1	2	2	1	1	-
Boyfriend/girlfriend	2	2	1	2	3	1	-
Friend	12	8	9	28	2	4	-
CPN/nurse	-	-	0	-	-	1	[1]
O.T	-	-	-	-	1	-	-
Social worker	0	-	1	-	2	-	-
Home careworker	0	5	0	2	-	2	[1]
Voluntary worker	0	1	1	2	3	2	-
Landlord landlady	0	-	-	-	-	-	-
Paid domestic help	5	8	-	-	-	2	-
Paid nurse	-	-	-	-	-	-	-
Bank manager	-	-	-	-	2	-	-
Solicitor	-	-	1	-	-	-	-
Other person	11	0	10	4	9	1	-
Base	*219*	*153*	*137*	*103*	*60*	*71*	*12*

* Percentages may add to more than 100% as some respondents had several helpers.

3   Recent stressful life events

3.1   Introduction

All adults interviewed in the survey were asked whether they had experienced each of 11 stressful life events during the past 6 months. The events and problems were taken from the previously developed List of Threatening Experiences[1]. They were:

1   Personally suffering a serious illness, injury or assault
2   A close relative suffering a serious illness, injury or assault
3   Death of a parent, spouse/partner, child, brother or sister
4   Death of a close family friend or another relative
5   Marital separation/ break-up of steady relationship
6   Serious problem with a close friend, neighbour or relative
7   Redundancy/ sacking from job
8   Unsuccessfully seeking work for more than one month
9   Major financial crisis, such as losing the equivalent of 3 months income
10 Problems with the police involving a court appearance
11 Something valued being lost or stolen

For each event a respondent had experienced, further questions were asked relating to the support available for coping with the problem - from both family and friends, and professionals.

This chapter looks at stressful life events in three ways:

- the number of stressful life events experienced

- which events were experienced

- what coping strategies were employed.

The first two of these are considered in relation to the CIS-R score and according to neurotic disorder. The coping strategies of adults with each life event are then investigated, comparing those with and without a neurotic disorder.

Although this chapter will describe associations, causality should not be inferred from these results; many of the events considered can be both a cause, and a result of psychiatric morbidity and we do not know whether the neurotic symptoms preceded the stressful life event. It has previously been shown (Report 2, Chapter 1) that many people with neurotic disorders had experienced the symptoms leading to the diagnosis of their disorder for periods in excess of six months, suggesting that for these people the disorder may have been present prior to the stressful life event happening. Moreover some life events may have been on-going, having begun more than 6 months ago, for example a serious illness.

The events considered in the survey do not cover every common stressful life event, excluding for example, moving house and having a baby. When looking at the number of stressful life events experienced it should be remembered that the events may not carry equal weight in terms of their psychological impact, and that some of the events are more likely to be found in combination than others; for example, redundancy and seeking work. Nevertheless, this selection of stressful life events, and the total number of life events experienced, have been shown to be meaningful measures[2] and the instrument had many advantages for this survey due to its brevity and ability to be used by interviewers without clinical training.

3.2 Stressful life events and CIS-R score

Just over half of all adults had experienced a stressful life event in the past 6 months; 32% had experienced one such event and 21% had experienced 2 or more.

While about a third of adults had experienced one stressful life event regardless of CIS-R score, there was a strong linear relationship between having higher CIS-R scores and the experience of more than one stressful life event; the proportions of adults with experience of 2 or more stressful life events ranged from 15% of those scoring 0-5 on the CIS-R, to 42% of those scoring 18 or above. Although there was no overall difference between men

and women in the number of stressful life events they experienced, among those with CIS-R scores of 12 or more, a higher proportion of men had experience of 2 or more stressful life events (44%) compared with women (35%). (*Table 3.1, figure 3.1*)

For each specific stressful life event, the proportion of adults having experienced the problem in the past 6 months increased by CIS-R score. The strongest associations were found with having a serious problem with a close friend, neighbour or relative, affecting 5% of those with CIS-R scores of 0-5 compared with 26% of those with CIS-R scores of 18 or more; marital separation or break-up of steady relationship (4% and 12% respectively) and financial crisis (3% and 16%). Events least associated with CIS-R score were either the death of a close relative or redundancy. This last finding may seem surprising, however a half of those losing their jobs within the past 6 months had also been re-employed within this period. (*Table 3.2*)

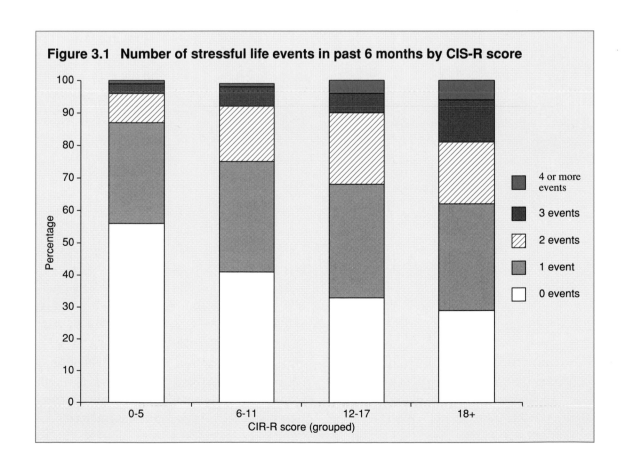

Figure 3.1 Number of stressful life events in past 6 months by CIS-R score

3.3 Stressful life events and neurotic disorders

Seventy one percent of adults with a neurotic disorder had experienced a recent stressful life event compared with 48% of those with no disorder. Those with depressive episode, OCD and phobia were most likely to have had a stressful life event; over three quarters of these adults had experienced at least one of the events, and over half of those with depressive episode had experienced 2 or more (compared with 17% of those with no disorder). *(Table 3.3)*

Almost half (49%) of adults with 2 or more neurotic disorders had experienced 2 or more stressful life events compared with just over a third (36%) of those with only one neurotic disorder. *(Table 3.4)*

For each life event considered, the proportion of adults with experience of the event was higher among adults with a neurotic disorder than among those with no neurotic disorder. The greatest differences were found for: serious problems with a close friend, having a serious personal illness, a financial crisis, and experiencing the break-up of a marriage or relationship.

The same relationships were found for each disorder, although their strength varied. Adults with depressive episode were most likely to have experienced many of the life events. *(Table 3.5)*

Particularly strong associations by disorder are shown in Figure 3.2.

Neurotic disorders among those with stressful life events

The relationship between stressful life events and neurotic disorders was also investigated by considering the proportion of adults with experience of each life event who were identified as having a neurotic disorder. Table 3.6 shows that a considerably higher proportion of adults with stressful life events had a neurotic

disorder compared with adults with no stressful life events; 26% of women and 18% of men with any stressful life event had a neurotic disorder compared with 13% and 7% respectively of those with no stressful life events. For some particular stressful life events, sex differences were more pronounced. For example, 20% of men who had lost a close relative in the past 6 months had a neurotic disorder, 3 times the proportion of those with no stressful life event. For women, the corresponding proportions were 26% compared with 13%, a ratio of 2:1.

Overall the strongest associations between stressful life events and the presence of a neurotic disorder were found for those experiencing problems with the police (39% had neurotic disorder), serious problems with a close friend (37%) and financial crisis (36%). The weakest relationships were for death and serious illness of relatives, redundancy and seeking work (20-23% of adults having experienced each of these had a neurotic disorder). *(Table 3.6, Figure 3.3)*

3.4 Coping with stressful life events

For each stressful life event experienced, people were asked whether anyone among their family or friends understood what the event felt like and if so, whether they could talk openly about it and get support and understanding. They were then asked whether they had received any professional help.

Most adults did have someone among their family and friends who could understand and help with each stressful life event. For most events, over three quarters of people affected received such help. Marital separation or the break up of a steady relationship and problems with the police were least likely to be understood by family and friends although around two thirds of adults still received help from this source. For many of the stressful life events a lower proportion of adults with neurotic disorders obtained help from family and friends compared with those with no disorder. However

Figure 3.2 Stressful life events strongly associated with neurotic disorders

Disorder	Recent Stressful life event strongly associated with disorder	Percentage of people experiencing life event	
		Those with a neurotic disorder	Those with no neurotic disorder
Generalised Anxiety Disorder	• Death of close family friend or other relative	24%	15%
	• Major financial crisis	18%	4%
Depressive Episode	• Serious personal illness	21%	4%
	• Break up of marriage/ relationship	14%	4%
	• Serious problem close friend	33%	7%
Phobia	• Serious problem with close friend	30%	7%
Obsessive Compulsive Disorder	• Serious illness of close relative	23%	12%
	• Serious problem with close friend	29%	7%
Panic disorder	• Death of close relative	3%	3%
	• Break up of marriage/ relationship	16%	4%

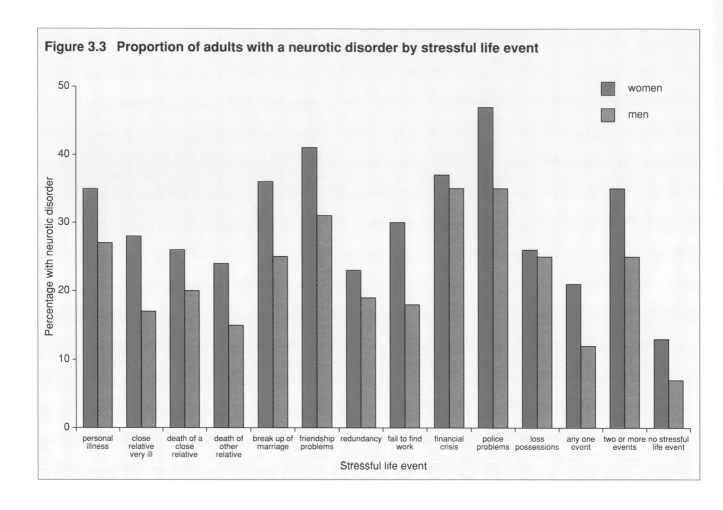

Figure 3.3 Proportion of adults with a neurotic disorder by stressful life event

this finding was statistically significant only for one of the most common stressful life events, the serious illness of a close relative (72% of those with a neurotic disorder received help from family and friends compared with 81% of those with no neurotic disorder).

A far smaller proportion of adults experiencing stressful life events received professional help than help from family or friends. There was greater variability in the proportions of people receiving help from professionals depending on the type of life event experienced. The proportions receiving such help ranged from 66% of those with a serious personal illness to 2% of those experiencing the death of a close relative. An indication of the type of help received ('practical' or 'someone to talk to') is given at the end of this section.

Adults received different levels of professional help according to whether they had a neurotic

disorder. For the bereavement and relationship problems, adults with a neurotic disorder were more likely than those with no disorder to receive professional help. Among those unsuccessfully seeking work, adults with a neurotic disorder were less likely to receive professional help than those without a disorder. There were no differences between the two groups in the proportions receiving professional help in coping with a financial crisis, police problems or the loss of valued possessions.

Most people receiving professional help had also had help from family and friends. (*Table 3.7*)

Those who had not received professional help were asked whether they had wanted such help, either practical assistance, or talking the problem over with a professional.
Thus, it is possible to classify all those who experienced a stressful life events in terms of

the type of professional help received or wanted:

Received help
Received practical professional help
Talked things over with a professional
Wanted help
Wanted practical professional help
Wanted to talk things over with a professional
Help not received and not wanted

For each life event, a higher proportion of adults with a neurotic disorder, compared with adults with no disorder, wanted help. For example, 9% of adults with a neurotic disorder wanted professional help in dealing with the breakdown of a relationship compared with 2% of those without a neurotic disorder and the corresponding proportions in relation to having a major financial crisis were 22% and 13%.

Whether people wanted practical assistance or to talk things over varied by type of stressful life event. Among adults with a neurotic disorder who wanted help to cope with redundancy or unsuccessful job seeking, the majority wanted practical help. Those who suffered a bereavement mostly wanted to talk this over with a professional. (*Table 3.8*)

3.5 Odds ratios of factors associated with having two or more stressful life events in the past 6 months

While this chapter has shown associations between stressful life events and the presence of a neurotic disorder, associations between socio-demographic or socio-economic characteristics and stressful life events have not yet

been considered. Multiple logistic regression was carried out to identify factors independently associated with having a stressful life event. Taking into account many socio-demographic and economic factors, the presence of a neurotic disorder was significantly positively associated with having experienced 2 or more stressful life events in the six months prior to interview. The odds of having 2 or more stressful life events were two and a half times higher among those with a neurotic disorder compared with those with no disorder.

One factor was more strongly associated with experiencing stressful life events than the presence of a neurotic disorder: employment status. The odds of having had 2 or more stressful life events in the last 6 months were almost 5 times higher among those who were unemployed compared with those working full-time. The very strong association with employment status is likely to reflect, at least in part, the fact that being made redundant and unsuccessfully seeking work for a period of one month or more were items on the list of stressful events. The full list of factors independently associated with having 2 or more stressful life events, and their odds, are shown in Table 3.9.

References

1 Brugha, T. S., Bebbington, P., Tennant, C. & Hurry, J. (1985). The List of Threatening Experiences: a subset of 12 life event categories with considerable long term contextual threat. *Psychological Medicine,* **15:** 189-194

2 Brugha, T. S. & Cragg, D. (1990) The list of threatening experiences: the reliability and validity of a brief life events questionnaire. *Acta Psychiatrica Scandinavica,* **82:** 77-81

Table 3.1 Number of stressful life events experienced in the last six months by CIS-R score and sex

Number of stressful life events	CIS-R score (grouped)						All
	0-5	6-11	12-17	18+	0-11	12+	
	%	%	%	%	%	%	%
Women							
0	56	41	33	29	52	31	48
1	31	34	35	33	32	34	32
2	9	17	22	19	11	20	13
3	3 ⌉13	6 ⌉25	6 ⌉32	13 ⌉39	4 ⌉16	10 ⌉35	5 ⌉19
4 or more	1	1	4	7	1	5	2
Any stressful life event	**44**	**59**	**67**	**71**	**48**	**69**	**52**
Base	*2917*	*1116*	*437*	*437*	*4034*	*874*	*4908*
Men							
0	53	38	29	21	50	25	48
1	30	32	32	30	31	31	31
2	12	18	23	28	13	26	14
3	4 ⌉17	7 ⌉29	10 ⌉39	12 ⌉49	4 ⌉19	11 ⌉44	5 ⌉22
4 or more	1	4	7	9	2	8	2
Any stressful life event	**47**	**62**	**71**	**79**	**50**	**75**	**52**
Base	*3539*	*773*	*265*	*256*	*4312*	*521*	*4833*
All adults							
0	54	40	31	26	51	29	48
1	31	33	34	32	31	33	32
2	11	18	22	22	12	22	14
3	3 ⌉15	6 ⌉26	7 ⌉35	13 ⌉42	4 ⌉18	10 ⌉39	5 ⌉21
4 or more	1	2	5	7	1	6	2
Any stressful life event	**46**	**60**	**69**	**74**	**49**	**71**	**52**
Base	*6456*	*1890*	*702*	*694*	*8346*	*1396*	*9741*

Table 3.2 Stressful life events experienced in the last six months by CIS-R score and sex

Type of stressful life event	CIS-R score (grouped)						All
	0-5	6-11	12-17	18+	0-11	12+	
	Percentage affected						
Death of other relative	14	18	20	19	15	19	16
Serious illness of close relative	11	16	19	20	12	20	13
Seeking work unsuccessfully	11	12	15	18	11	16	12
Serious problem with close friend	5	12	18	26	7	22	9
Valuable possessions lost/stolen	6	8	10	12	6	11	7
Serious personal illness	4	8	8	14	5	10	6
Major financial crisis	3	7	10	16	4	11	5
Break-up of marriage/relationship	4	7	9	12	4	10	5
Made redundant from job	4	4	6	6	4	6	4
Death of close relative	3	4	4	5	3	4	3
Problems with police-court	1	2	4	4	1	4	2
Any of above	**46**	**60**	**69**	**74**	**49**	**71**	**52**
Base	*6456*	*1890*	*702*	*694*	*8346*	*1396*	*9741*

Table 3.3 Number of stressful life events by neurotic disorder

Number of stressful life events	Mixed anxiety and depressive disorder	Generalised Anxiety Disorder	Depressive episode	Phobia	Obsessive-Compulsive Disorder	Panic disorder	Any neurotic disorder	No neurotic disorder
	%	%	%	%	%	%	%	%
0	31	26	18	24	23	28	29	52
1	34	33	30	36	30	33	33	31
2	23	22	24	17	22	23	22	12
3	7 ⎫ 35	11 ⎫ 40	17 ⎫ 52	13 ⎫ 40	14 ⎫ 47	9 ⎫ 39	10 ⎫ 38	4 ⎫ 17
4 or more	4 ⎭	8 ⎭	12 ⎭	10 ⎭	10 ⎭	7 ⎭	7 ⎭	1 ⎭
Any stressful life event	**69**	**74**	**82**	**76**	**77**	**72**	**71**	**48**
Base	*750*	*439*	*220*	*180*	*157*	*93*	*1557*	*8184*

51

Table 3.4 Number of stressful life events by number of neurotic disorders

Number of stressful life events	No neurotic disorder	One neurotic disorder	Two or more neurotic disorders
	%	%	%
0	51	31	16
1	31	32	35
2	12 ⎤ 17	22 ⎤ 36	23 ⎤ 49
3	4	9	16
4 or more	1	6	11
Any stressful life event	**69**	**84**	**49**
Base	*8184*	*1348*	*209*

Table 3.5 The proportion of adults with each stressful life event by neurotic disorder

Type of stressful life event	Mixed anxiety and depressive disorder	Generalised Anxiety Disorder	Depressive episode	Phobia	Obsessive-Compulsive Disorder	Panic disorder	Any neurotic disorder	No neurotic disorder	All
	Percentage affected								
Death of other relative	20	24	19	22	16	13	19	15	16
Serious illness of close relative	20	19	22	22	23	18	19	12	13
Seeking work unsuccessfully	15	18	19	19	21	13	17	11	12
Serious problem with close friend	17	24	33	30	29	27	21	7	9
Valuable possessions lost/stolen	9	13	17	14	15	9	11	6	7
Serious personal illness	8	12	21	16	17	9	11	4	6
Major financial crisis	9	18	17	8	15	12	11	4	5
Break up of marriage/relationship	9	9	14	10	14	16	10	4	5
Made redundant from job	6	5	6	5	3	4	6	4	4
Death of close relative	5	3	6	5	8	4	5	3	3
Problems with police - court	4	4	4	5	4	3	4	1	2
Any of above	**69**	**74**	**82**	**76**	**77**	**72**	**71**	**48**	**52**
Base	*750*	*439*	*220*	*180*	*157*	*93*	*1557*	*8184*	*9741*

Table 3.6 Presence of a neurotic disorder by stressful life events and sex

	Death of other relative	Serious illness of close relative	Seeking work unsuccessfully	Serious problem with close friend	Valuable possessions lost/stolen	Serious personal illness
	%	%	%	%	%	%
Women						
Neurotic disorder	24	28	30	41	26	35
No neurotic disorder	76	72	70	59	74	65
Base	*821*	*730*	*418*	*532*	*336*	*250*
Men						
Neurotic disorder	15	17	18	31	25	27
No neurotic disorder	85	83	82	69	75	73
Base	*707*	*575*	*729*	*356*	*341*	*288*
All adults						
Neurotic disorder	20	23	22	37	26	31
No neurotic disorder	80	77	78	63	75	69
Base	*1528*	*1605*	*1147*	*889*	*677*	*538*

Table 3.6 Presence of a neurotic disorder by stressful life events and sex - *continued*

	Major financial crisis	Break up of marriage relationship	Made redundant from job	Death of a close relative	Problems with police - court	Any stressful life event	No stressful life event
	%	%	%	%	%	%	%
Women							
Neurotic disorder	37	36	23	26	47	26	13
No neurotic disorder	63	64	77	74	53	74	87
Base	*213*	*260*	*136*	*168*	*52*	*2534*	*2375*
Men							
Neurotic disorder	35	25	19	20	35	18	7
No neurotic disorder	65	75	81	80	65	82	93
Base	*278*	*260*	*287*	*150*	*113*	*2539*	*2294*
All adults							
Neurotic disorder	36	30	21	23	39	52	10
No neurotic disorder	64	70	79	77	61	48	90
Base	*491*	*520*	*423*	*318*	*165*	*3970*	*4214*

Table 3.7 The receipt of help from family and friends and professionals by stressful life events and the presence or absence of a neurotic disorder

Adults with each type of stressful life event

Types of stressful life events	Help received	Any neurotic disorder	No neurotic disorder	All adults
		Percentage receiving help		
Death of other relative	from family and friends only	76 ⎱ 80	85 ⎱ 87	84 ⎱ 86
	from family and professionals	3 ⎰ 4	2 ⎰ 2	2 ⎰ 2
	from professionals only	1	0	0
	Base	*301*	*1234*	*1535*
Serious illness of close relative	from family and friends only	60 ⎱ 72	69 ⎱ 81	67 ⎱ 79
	from family and professionals	12 ⎰ 15	12 ⎰ 16	12 ⎰ 16
	from professionals only	3	4	4
	Base	*300*	*1010*	*1309*
Seeking work unsuccessfully	from family and friends only	52 ⎱ 70	53 ⎱ 79	53 ⎱ 77
	from family and professionals	18 ⎰ 23	26 ⎰ 32	24 ⎰ 30
	from professionals only	5	6	6
	Base	*259*	*892*	*1151*
Serious problem with close friend	from family and friends only	50 ⎱ 67	66 ⎱ 78	60 ⎱ 74
	from family and professionals	17 ⎰ 24	12 ⎰ 15	14 ⎰ 18
	from professionals only	7	3	4
	Base	*334*	*568*	*902*
Valuable possessions lost or stolen	from family and friends only	59 ⎱ 76	70 ⎱ 86	67 ⎱ 83
	from family and professionals	17 ⎰ 21	16 ⎰ 19	16 ⎰ 19
	from professionals only	4	3	3
	Base	*173*	*509*	*682*
Serious personal illness	from family and friends only	27 ⎱ 66	26 ⎱ 78	26 ⎱ 74
	from family and professionals	39 ⎰ 59	52 ⎰ 69	48 ⎰ 66
	from professionals only	20	17	18
	Base	*167*	*374*	*541*
Major financial crisis	from family and friends only	55 ⎱ 72	59 ⎱ 79	56 ⎱ 76
	from family and professionals	20 ⎰ 22	20 ⎰ 23	20 ⎰ 23
	from professionals only	2	3	3
	Base	*177*	*318*	*495*
Break-up of marriage/ relationship	from family and friends only	54 ⎱ 65	58 ⎱ 65	57 ⎱ 65
	from family and professionals	11 ⎰ 15	7 ⎰ 10	8 ⎰ 11
	from professionals only	4	3	3
	Base	*160*	*369*	*529*

Table 3.7   The receipt of help from family and friends and professionals by stressful life events and the presence or absence of a neurotic disorder - *continued*

Adults with each type of stressful life event

Types of stressful life events	Help received	Any neurotic disorder		No neurotic disorder		All adults	
		Percentage receiving help					
Made redundant from job	from family and friends only	54	65	61	74	59	72
	from family and professionals	11		13		13	
	from professionals only	4	15	3	16	3	16
	Base	*88*		*342*		*429*	
Death of close relative	from family and friends only	65	81	79	86	64	85
	from family and professionals	16		7		9	
	from professionals only	5	21	3	10	4	13
	Base	*74*		*251*		*325*	
Problems with police-court	from family and friends only	38	63	44	64	42	64
	from family and professionals	25		20		22	
	from professionals only	8	33	11	31	10	32
	Base	*64*		*107*		*171*	

55

Table 3.8 The receipt of professional help by stressful life events and the presence or absence of a neurotic disorder

Adults with each type of stressful life event

Types of stressful life events	Types of professional help received, or wanted, but not received*	Any neurotic disorder	No neurotic disorder	All Adults
		~ %	~ %	~ %
Death of other relative	received practical help	1 ⎤ 3	0 ⎤ 1	0 ⎤ 2
	had someone to talk to	3 ⎦	1 ⎦	2 ⎦
	wanted practical help	0 ⎤ 2	0 ⎤ 0	0 ⎤ 1
	wanted someone to talk to	2 ⎦	0 ⎦	1 ⎦
	did not want any help	95	98	98
	Base	*301*	*1227*	*1528*
Serious illness of close relative	received practical help	9 ⎤ 14	10 ⎤ 15	10 ⎤ 15
	had someone to talk to	9 ⎦	10 ⎦	9 ⎦
	wanted practical help	2 ⎤ 8	1 ⎤ 2	1 ⎤ 3
	wanted someone to talk to	7 ⎦	1 ⎦	3 ⎦
	did not want any help	78	83	82
	Base	*299*	*1006*	*1305*
Seeking work unsuccessfully	received practical help	19 ⎤ 23	27 ⎤ 32	25 ⎤ 30
	had someone to talk to	11 ⎦	13 ⎦	13 ⎦
	wanted practical help	12 ⎤ 15	5 ⎤ 6	6 ⎤ 8
	wanted someone to talk to	7 ⎦	4 ⎦	4 ⎦
	did not want any help	62	62	62
	Base	*259*	*889*	*1147*
Serious problem with close friend	received practical help	14 ⎤ 23	10 ⎤ 14	12 ⎤ 18
	had someone to talk to	15 ⎦	8 ⎦	11 ⎦
	wanted practical help	4 ⎤ 8	1 ⎤ 3	2 ⎤ 5
	wanted someone to talk to	6 ⎦	2 ⎦	4 ⎦
	did not want any help	69	82	77
	Base	*331*	*557*	*889*
Valuable possessions lost/ stolen	received practical help	16 ⎤ 20	14 ⎤ 18	15 ⎤ 18
	had someone to talk to	6 ⎦	6 ⎦	6 ⎦
	wanted practical help	5 ⎤ 7	1 ⎤ 2	2 ⎤ 3
	wanted someone to talk to	4 ⎦	0 ⎦	1 ⎦
	did not want any help	73	80	78
	Base	*173*	*504*	*677*
Serious personal illness	received practical help	45 ⎤ 59	60 ⎤ 69	55 ⎤ 66
	had someone to talk to	28 ⎦	27 ⎦	27 ⎦
	wanted practical help	4 ⎤ 7	1 ⎤ 2	2 ⎤ 3
	wanted someone to talk to	4 ⎦	1 ⎦	2 ⎦
	did not want any help	34	30	31
	Base	*166*	*371*	*538*

Table 3.8 The receipt of professional help by stressful life events and the presence or absence of a neurotic disorder - *continued*

Adults with each type of stressful life event

Types of stressful life events	Types of professional help received, or wanted, but not received*	Any neurotic disorder	No neurotic disorder	All adults
		~ %	~ %	~ %
Major financial crisis	received practical help	19 ⎤ 22	20 ⎤ 23	19 ⎤ 23
	had someone to talk to	12 ⎦	8 ⎦	9 ⎦
	wanted practical help	18 ⎤ 22	10 ⎤ 13	13 ⎤ 16
	wanted someone to talk to	12 ⎦	6 ⎦	8 ⎦
	did not want any help	56	64	61
	Base	*177*	*314*	*491*
Break up of marriage/ relationship	received practical help	6 ⎤ 15	4 ⎤ 10	5 ⎤ 12
	had someone to talk to	13 ⎦	8 ⎦	9 ⎦
	wanted practical help	3 ⎤ 9	1 ⎤ 2	2 ⎤ 4
	wanted someone to talk to	8 ⎦	2 ⎦	4 ⎦
	did not want any help	76	88	84
	Base	*159*	*361*	*520*
Made redundant from job	received practical help	10 ⎤ 15	15 ⎤ 16	14 ⎤ 16
	had someone to talk to	8 ⎦	8 ⎦	8 ⎦
	wanted practical help	6 ⎤ 12	1 ⎤ 3	2 ⎤ 5
	wanted someone to talk to	7 ⎦	3 ⎦	4 ⎦
	did not want any help	72	80	79
	Base	*88*	*336*	*423*
Death of close relative	received practical help	8 ⎤ 22	4 ⎤ 10	5 ⎤ 13
	had someone to talk to	21 ⎦	9 ⎦	12 ⎦
	wanted practical help	- ⎤ 8	1 ⎤ 1	1 ⎤ 2
	wanted someone to talk to	8 ⎦	- ⎦	2 ⎦
	did not want any help	70	89	85
	Base	*74*	*244*	*318*
Problems with police - court	received practical help	21 ⎤ 33	26 ⎤ 31	24 ⎤ 32
	had someone to talk to	23 ⎦	16 ⎦	19 ⎦
	wanted practical help	6 ⎤ 8	3 ⎤ 6	4 ⎤ 7
	wanted someone to talk to	4 ⎦	6 ⎦	5 ⎦
	did not want any help	59	63	62
	Base	*64*	*101*	*165*

~ The total percentages in these columns exceed 100% as some people received or wanted both types of help

* Those described as wanting help include people who tried to get professional help but who did not obtain it, and those who did not try to get professional help because they did not know where to get it from

Table 3. 9   Odds ratios of neurotic disorder and socio-demographic correlates of having two or more stressful life events

		Adjusted O.R	95% C.I
Neurotic disorder	No neurotic disorder	1.00	....
	Neurotic disorder	2.56**	(2.25-2.91)
Long-standing physical illness	No physical complaint	1.00	....
	Physical complaint	1.43**	(1.28-1.61)
Sex	Men	1.00	....
	Women	0.89*	(0.79-1.00)
Age	16-24	1.00	....
	25-34	0.75**	(0.62-0.90)
	35-44	0.83	(0.68-1.02)
	45-54	0.69**	(0.56-0.85)
	55-64	0.50**	(0.40-0.63)
Family unit type	Couple, no children	1.00	....
	Couple & children	1.09	(0.94-1.27)
	Lone parent and child(ren)	1.48**	(1.17-1.89)
	One person only	1.22*	(1.02-1.45)
	Adult with parents	1.21	(0.96-1.53)
	Adult with parent	1.09	(0.65-1.24)
Qualifications	A level or higher	1.00	....
	GCSE/ O level	0.97	(0.85-1.12)
	Other	1.00	(0.83-1.20)
	None	0.80**	(0.69-0.93)
Employment status	Working full-time	1.00	....
	Working part-time	1.00	(0.84-1.18)
	Unemployed	4.83**	(4.10-5.70)
	Economically inactive	1.05	(0.90-1.22)
Type of accomodation	Detached	1.00	....
	Semi-detached	0.99	(0.84-1.15)
	Terraced	1.25*	(1.07-1.47)
	Flat	1.43**	(1.18-1.72)

Other factors included in the regression analysis, but found not to be independently associated with having 2 or more stressful life events were: ethnicity, type of occupation and locality.

* $p < 0.05$ ** $p < 0.01$

4   Social functioning

4.1   Introduction

This survey considered three aspects of social functioning:

- self-perceived social support
- extent of social networks
- involvement in social and leisure activities

Questions to assess each of the above were asked of all survey respondents.

The chapter begins by considering each aspect of social functioning in turn, and then looks at inter-relationships between the three main measures used. Differential use of services according to levels of social support is examined in the final section.

4.2   Perceived social support

Perceived social support was assessed from respondents' answers to 7 questions taken from the 1987 Health and Lifestyle survey[1]; these questions were also asked in the Health Survey for England[2], providing additional comparative data. The seven questions take the form of statements which individuals could say were not true, partly true, or certainly true of their family and friends. Scores of 1- 3 were obtained for each question and overall scores ranged from 7 to 21. The maximum score of 21 indicated no lack of social support, scores of 18 to 20 indicated a moderate lack of social support and scores of 17 and below showed that individuals perceived a severe lack of social support. The seven questions are:

There are people I know - amongst my family or friends -
1) who do things to make me happy

2) who make me feel loved
3) who can be relied on no matter what happens
4) who would see that I am taken care of if I needed to be
5) who accept me just as I am
6) who make me feel an important part of their lives
7) who give me support and encouragement

In this survey, 69% of women and 59% of men reported no lack of social support. As well as differences by sex, variation was evident for people of different ages (with those in the youngest age group most likely to perceive a lack of social support). Compared with the findings of the Health Survey for England, a smaller proportion of respondents to this survey reported a severe lack of social support (9% compared with 14% overall). This difference may be a result of the data being collected in different ways on the two surveys; interviewers asked the questions on the psychiatric morbidity survey, while responses were entered in a self-completion booklet by respondents in the Health Survey. It is possible that people felt more inclined to indicate 'not true' to the statements when written down, in private, than when read out by an interviewer. (*Table 4.1*)

Data from the psychiatric morbidity survey have shown considerable variation in psychiatric morbidity according to marital status and family unit types (Reports 1 and 2[3, 4]). Part of the explanation for this might be the differing levels of social support associated with different circumstances. Larger proportions of adults living with a lone parent, and of people living alone or as lone parents with children, reported a severe lack of social support compared with adults living in couples. Single, divorced and separated people were most likely to lack social support. For example, 13% of divorced people perceived a severe lack of social support, compared with 8% of those who were married. (*Tables 4.2 and 4.3*)

The relationship between psychiatric morbidity and perceived social support

The proportion of people who felt a severe lack of social support increased with CIS-R score, from 8% of those scoring 0-5, to 21% of those with a score of 18 or more. Among adults scoring 0-17, a higher proportion of men perceived a lack of social support compared with women; however, among those with scores of 18 or more on the CIS-R there was no difference in perception of social support between the sexes. The proportion of women classified as having a severe lack of social support jumped from 12% of those scoring 12-17 on the CIS-R to 21% of those scoring 18 or more. (*Table 4.4*)

Adults with phobia and depressive episode were most likely to report a lack of social support; over half of those with these disorders (phobia, 56% and depressive episode, 53%) felt some lack of social support compared with 34% of those with no neurotic disorder. A higher proportion of adults with 2 or more neurotic disorders perceived a severe lack of social support (26%) than among those with just one neurotic disorder (16%) or no neurotic disorder (8%). (*Tables 4.5 and 4.6*)

The relationship between psychiatric morbidity and social support may also be considered by looking at the proportion of people with a neurotic disorder according to the level of social support they reported. The proportion of adults with a neurotic disorder among the group with a severe lack of social support (29%), was double that of the group with no lack (14%). (*Table 4.7*)

For adults with each level of perceived social support, the proportion with a neurotic disorder increased with the number of stressful life events[5] experienced in the last 6 months.

Looking at the extremes, 9% of those with no lack of social support and no stressful life events had a neurotic disorder, compared with 46% of those with a severe lack of social support and experience of 2 or more stressful life events. It is interesting to note that those with no lack of social support and experience of 2 or more stressful life events, were *more* likely to have a neurotic disorder than adults with a severe lack of social support and no stressful life events (26% compared with 18%). (*Table 4.8*)

4.3   Extent of social networks

In this survey information about social networks focused on the numbers of friends and relatives (aged 16 and over) respondents felt close to.

Data were collected about three groups of people:

1) *adults who lived with respondents that respondents felt close to*
2) *relatives who did not live with respondents that they felt close to*
3) *friends or acquaintances who did not live with respondents that would be described as close or good friends.*

Close friends and relatives form an individual's 'primary support group'. Previous research has suggested that adults with a total primary support group of 3 people or fewer are at greatest risk of psychiatric morbidity[6,7].

For most analysis in this section, the size of the primary support group including people from all groups above, has been divided into three categories (0-3, 4-8, 9 or more). Individuals for whom the size of the primary support group could not be calculated because of missing data (about 1% of the total sample), have been grouped with those having 0-3 people in their primary support group; a high proportion of people in this group had a neurotic disorder, and it is hypothesised, and supported by comments from interviewers, that these questions may have been omitted in some cases because they were upsetting to informants with small social networks.

Like perceived social support, the size of primary support group varied by family unit type. Most adults had a primary support group of 9 or more (61%), but less than half the lone parents (42%) and adults living with one parent (46%) had primary support groups of this size. The proportion of people with primary support groups of 3 or fewer, ranged from 5% of couples without children to 14% of lone parents. (*Table 4.9*)

The relationship between social network size and psychiatric morbidity

The number of people that respondents felt close to varied for adults with and without a neurotic disorder. Those with disorders were more likely to live alone (18% compared with 11%), and if they did not live alone, they were more likely to feel close to none of the people they lived with (5% compared with 2%). Forty one per cent of adults with a neurotic disorder had no more than 2 relatives they felt close to outside the household; this compares with less than a third (31%) of adults with no neurotic disorder. Looking at the number of friends outside the household that people felt close to, the same pattern was found; 37% of those with a neurotic disorder had less than three close friends, compared with 25% of those with no disorder. (*Table 4.10*)

The proportion of adults with a primary support group of 3 people or fewer increased by CIS-R score, although there was no difference between those scoring 0-5 and those scoring 6-11 (6%). Nine per cent of adults with CIS-R scores of 12-17 had a primary support group of 0-3 and this rose to 17% of those with scores of 18 or more. (*Table 4.11*)

Those with phobia, depressive episode and obsessive-compulsive disorder were most likely to have the smallest primary support groups; 21%, 20% and 19% respectively, compared with 6% among those with no neurotic disorder. While 11% of adults with one neurotic disorder had a primary support group of 3 or fewer individuals, the corresponding proportion among those with two or more neurotic disorders rose to 21%. (*Tables 4.12 and 4.13*)

Considering the prevalence of a neurotic disorder according to the size of primary support group, variations are very clear. For both women and men, the prevalence of neurotic disorders among those with a primary support group of 9 or more, was less than half that among those with a primary support group of 3 or fewer. For example, 15% of women in the former group had a neurotic disorder compared with 36% of those with a primary support group of just 0-3 people. (*Table 4.14*)

Almost half the adults with a primary support group of 3 people or fewer, who had experienced 2 or more stressful life events in the last 6 months, had a neurotic disorder (47%). This compared with 18% of those with the same size social network, but no stressful life events. A quarter of those who had experienced 2 or more recent stressful life events but had primary support groups of 9 or more had a neurotic disorder. (*Table 4.15*)

Multiple logistic regression

Multiple logistic regression was carried out to see how the odds of having a small primary support group were associated with having a neurotic disorder, controlling for various socio-demographic factors. The presence of a neurotic disorder was found to be significantly independently associated with having a small primary support group; the odds of having a primary support group of 3 people or fewer was two times higher among those with a disorder compared with those with no neurotic disorder. (*Table 4.16*)

Logistic regression was also employed to investigate perceived social support. Both the presence of a neurotic disorder, and the size of primary support group were independently associated with perceiving a severe lack of social support, controlling for socio-demographic factors. Although those with neurotic disorders were more likely to have a small support network, this analysis shows that they also perceived their social support network, whatever its size, to be less supportive than did those without a neurotic disorder. Whether there was an actual difference in quality, or just a perceptual difference is unknown. Other characteristics with strong independent associations with perceiving a severe lack of social support were being female or being a lone parent. (*Table 4.17*)

4.4 Social and leisure activities

All survey respondents were asked about the activities they did both in and out of the home during their leisure time. The lists of activities used in the survey were developed specifically for this project: nine activities in the home and fifteen out of the home were asked about. In this section, participation in specific activities in and out of the home is first considered, followed by a measure of the total number of leisure time activities respondents participated in; the number of activities are grouped as follows: 0-3, 4-9, 10 or more; these groupings were chosen because of their relationship with having a neurotic disorder.

The relationship between leisure activities and psychiatric morbidity

For about half of the activities selected, the proportions of people participating in the activity varied significantly by CIS-R score. Even for activities where differences were not significant, there was a general tendency for participation to fall off with increasing CIS-R score. Comparing rates of participation among those scoring 0-11 and those scoring 12 or more on the CIS-R, those activities which

showed significant variation are listed below; starred items varied most markedly.

In and around the home:	*Out of the home:*
TV / radio	Going to pubs and
Reading books/	restaurants *
newspapers	Going for a walk
Gardening *	Participation in sports *
Games	Cinema, theatre,
DIY / car	concerts *
maintenance *	Clubs, organisations *
	Sports as a spectator *
	Church

For example, half of those with a CIS-R score of 0-11 participated in sports compared with just over a third of those with a CIS-R score of 12 or more (35%). (*Table 4.18*)

Participation in activities varied considerably among those with different neurotic disorders, partly serving to confound the analysis by CIS-R score. Those with depressive episode and phobia tended to have the lowest levels of participation, while those with panic disorder had higher rates of participation in many activities.

Leisure activities in and around the home

Compared with others, people with depressive episode were least likely to spend their time reading books or newspapers, entertaining friends and relatives, or pursuing hobbies. For example, 41% of those with depressive episode entertained friends and relatives, compared with 56% of those with no neurotic disorder. Those with phobia were least likely to garden, possibly due to specific isolated phobias involving insects and birds, and to agoraphobia (22% of those with phobia gardened compared with 46% of those with no neurotic disorder). People with panic disorder appeared more likely to spend their time pursuing hobbies (43% compared with 34% of those with no disorder) although this difference was not statistically significant.

Leisure activities out of the home

Only 40% of people with phobia went for a walk and only 52% went to pubs and restaurants compared with 54% and 70% respectively of those with no neurotic disorder; those with social phobia or agoraphobia may find such activities particularly difficult. It is interesting to note that while similar proportions of adults with panic disorder and no disorder were involved in most activities, this was not the case for participation in sports where those with panic disorder were more similar to adults with other neurotic disorders. (*Table 4.19*)

Total number of leisure activities

Women and men were involved in similar numbers of leisure activities; most (56%) participated in 4-9 activities while 38% were involved in 10 or more, and only 6% were involved in 3 or fewer activities. The proportion of people involved in 3 or fewer activities increased with CIS-R score; from 5% among those scoring 0-5, to 16% of those scoring 18 or more. (*Table 4.20*)

People with depressive episode were four times more likely to participate in 0-3 activities than those with no neurotic disorder (21% compared with 5%). The proportion of adults with panic disorder participating in 0-3 activities (5%) was the same as among those with no neurotic disorder. While 40% of people with no neurotic disorder had 10 or more leisure pursuits, the corresponding figures for those with one, and with two or more neurotic disorders, were 30% and 18% respectively. (*Tables 4.21 and 4.22*)

Looking at the data from a different angle, an almost linear progression was found in the proportion of people with a neurotic disorder according to the number of leisure activities they participated in. While only 12% of those spending time on 10 or more activities had a disorder, the figures rose to 20% of those

involved in 4-9 activities and 30% of those recording only 0-3 activities. (*Table 4.23*)

4.5 Relationships between the measures of social functioning

Perceived social support and size of primary support group

The size of an individual's primary support group might be considered likely to be closely related to the individual's perceived social support. Certainly the two are related, however, it is surprising to find that over a quarter of those with the largest primary support groups perceived a lack of social support, and to see that almost a third (29%) of those with a primary support group of 3 people or fewer felt no lack of social support. (*Table 4.24*)

Not surprisingly, the prevalence of neurotic disorders was highest among the group who felt a severe lack of social support, and had a primary support group of 3 people or less (41% had a disorder). It is interesting to see that neurotic disorders affected similar proportions of people among the group with a severe lack of social support, but a large primary support group (21% had a disorder), and the group perceiving no lack of social support, but having the smallest primary support group (24% had a disorder). (*Table 4.25*)

Primary support group and participation in leisure activities

People who had large primary support groups also tended to participate in a larger number of leisure activities; 45% of those with 9 or more people in their primary support group recorded 10 or more leisure activities, compared with 16% of those with the smallest primary support groups. (*Table 4.26*)

Thirty-five per cent of adults with a primary support group of 3 people or fewer, and who were involved in the smallest number of activities (0-3) had a neurotic disorder, compared with 10% of the group who had the largest primary support groups and the most leisure interests. (*Table 4.27*)

Perceived social support and participation in leisure activities

The number of activities people were involved in declined as the lack of perceived social support increased; 43% of adults with no lack of social support were involved in 10 or more activities compared with 33% of those with a moderate, and 21% of those with a severe, lack of social support. (*Table 4.28*)

While only 10% of adults with no lack of social support, who participated in 10 or more leisure activities, had a neurotic disorder, the proportion rose to 23% of those with a severe lack of social support involved in 10 or more activities. This was identical to the proportion of those with no lack of social support who reported 3 or fewer leisure time activities. (*Tables 4.29*)

4.6 Social functioning and use of services

In coping with a given situation, it might be considered likely that an individual with a supportive social network would have less need for formal services than one with a lack of social support. This hypothesis is difficult to investigate due to the many different factors involved in obtaining services. Some analysis was undertaken among those with a neurotic disorder, to compare contact with a GP, receipt of counselling or therapy and receipt of professional help in coping with stressful life events for individuals with different levels of perceived social support.

Adults who felt they had a severe lack of social support were more likely to have contacted a GP in the last 12 months for a mental, nervous or emotional problem than those who reported no lack of social support (43% compared with 32%). However, it should be remembered that this does not take account of the fact, already shown in this

chapter, that those with a lack of social support had more severe neurotic disorders than those with no lack of social support. Receipt of counselling or therapy also appeared to vary by levels of social support. Overall, 9% of adults with a neurotic disorder had received some form of counselling. Among those perceiving a severe lack of social support the proportion was 13% compared with 7% among those reporting no lack of social support. There were no notable differences in receipt of professional help associated with stressful life events by levels of social support. (*Table 4.30*)

Notes and references

1   *The Health and Lifestyle Survey,* Health Promotion Research Trust, 1987

2   Breeze, E., Maidment, A., Bennett, N., Flatley, J., Carey, S. (1994) *Health Survey for England 1992,* HMSO, London: Table 2.27.

3   Meltzer, H., Gill, B., Petticrew, M., Hinds, K., (1995) *OPCS Surveys of Psychiatric Morbidity in Great Britain. Report 1: The prevalence of psychiatric morbidity among adults living in private households,* HMSO, London

4   Meltzer, H., Gill, B., Petticrew, M., Hinds, K., (1995) *OPCS Surveys of Psychiatric Morbidity in Great Britain. Report 2: Physical illness, service use and treatment of adults with psychiatric disorders,* HMSO, London

5   For details of the recent stressful life events included, see Chapter 3 of this report.

6   Brugha, T. S., Wing, J. K., Brewin, C. R., MacCarthy, B. & Lesage, A. (1993). The relationship of social network deficits with deficits in social functioning in long-term psychiatric disorders. *Social Psychiatry and Psychiatric Epidemiology,* **28,** 218-224

7   Brugha, T. S., Sturt, E., MacCarthy, B., Potter, J. Wykes, T. & Bebbington, P. E. (1987). The Interview Measure of Social Relationships: the description and evaluation of a survey instrument for assessing personal social resources. *Social Psychiatry,* **22,** 123-128

Table 4.1   Perceived social support by age and sex: comparison with Health Survey data

Perceived social support	Age											
	16-24		25-34		35-44		45-54		55-64		All *	
	PMS	HS	PMS	HS	PMS	HS	PMS	HS	PMS	HS	PMS	HS
	%	%	%	%	%	%	%	%	%	%	%	%
Women												
No lack	61	56	68	61	70	61	74	58	74	63	69	61
Moderate lack	28	32	23	27	23	25	20	29	20	27	23	27
Severe lack	11	12	8	12	7	14	6	13	6	10	8	12
Base	*917*	*523*	*1211*	*730*	*1057*	*683*	*929*	*537*	*784*	*495*	*4908*	*3806*
Men												
No lack	52	45	58	51	62	56	61	52	63	54	59	52
Moderate lack	35	36	31	34	28	31	28	32	27	28	30	32
Severe lack	13	19	10	15	10	13	10	16	11	18	11	16
Base	*947*	*430*	*1219*	*628*	*1000*	*614*	*915*	*517*	*753*	*434*	*4833*	*3297*
All adults												
No lack	56	51	63	56	66	59	68	55	68	59	64	57
Moderate lack	32	34	27	30	26	28	24	31	23	28	26	29
Severe lack	12	15	10	13	9	13	8	14	9	14	9	14
Base	*1864*	*993*	*2439*	*1358*	*2056*	*1297*	*1844*	*1054*	*1537*	*929*	*9741*	*7103*

* 'All' figures for the Health Survey (HS) include adults aged 16-100 while those for the Psychiatric Morbidity Survey (PMS) include only those aged 16-64. The pattern for HS respondents aged 65 and over was not very different from the pattern for younger adults so this difference should not bias the data.

Table 4.2 Perceived social support by family unit type and sex

| Perceived social support | Family unit type | | | | | | |
	Couple, no child(ren)	Couple & child(ren)	Lone parent & child(ren)	One person only	Adult with parents	Adult with one parent	All
	%	%	%	%	%	%	%
Women							
No lack	74	72	59	67	61	53	69
Moderate lack	21	22	29	22	29	34	23
Severe lack	6	7	12	10	10	13	8
Base	*1345*	*1942*	*494*	*592*	*419*	*115*	*4908*
Men							
No lack	65	62	57	52	52	41	59
Moderate lack	26	29	32	31	36	42	30
Severe lack	9	9	10	17	12	17	11
Base	*1236*	*1960*	*62*	*716*	*656*	*204*	*4833*
All adults							
No lack	70	67	59	59	56	45	64
Moderate lack	23	25	29	27	33	39	26
Severe lack	7	8	12	14	11	16	9
Base	*2581*	*3902*	*556*	*1308*	*1075*	*319*	*9741*

Table 4.3 Perceived social support by marital status

| Perceived social support | Marital status | | | | | | |
	Married	Cohabiting	Single	Widowed	Divorced	Separated	All
	%	%	%	%	%	%	%
All adults							
No lack	68	64	55	74	57	61	64
Moderate lack	24	28	32	16	29	25	26
Severe lack	8	8	13	10	13	14	9
Base	*5772*	*684*	*2344*	*211*	*502*	*182*	*9741*

Table 4.4 Perceived social support by CIS-R score

| Perceived social support | CIS-R score (grouped) | | | | | | |
	0 - 5	6-11	12-17	18+	0-11	12+	All
	%	%	%	%	%	%	%
Women							
No lack	73	67	68	48	72	58	69
Moderate lack	21	26	10	31	23	25	23
Severe lack	6	7	12	21	6	17	8
Base	*2917*	*1116*	*437*	*437*	*4034*	*874*	*4908*
Men							
No lack	61	56	53	45	60	49	59
Moderate lack	29	33	30	35	30	33	30
Severe lack	10	11	17	20	10	18	11
Base	*3539*	*773*	*265*	*256*	*4312*	*521*	*4833*
All adults							
No lack	67	62	62	47	66	56	64
Moderate lack	25	29	24	32	26	28	26
Severe lack	8	8	14	21	8	18	9
Base	*6456*	*1890*	*702*	*694*	*8346*	*1396*	*9741*

Table 4.5 Perceived social support by neurotic disorder

Perceived social support	Mixed anxiety and depressive disorder	Generalised Anxiety disorder	Depressive episode	Phobia	Obsessive-compulsive disorder	Panic disorder	Any neurotic disorder	No neurotic disorder
	%	%	%	%	%	%	%	%
All adults								
No lack	59	52	47	44	53	60	55	66
Moderate lack	27	27	28	31	25	24	28	26
Severe lack	14	21	25	25	22	16	17	8
Base	*750*	*439*	*220*	*180*	*157*	*93*	*1557*	*8184*

Table 4.6 Perceived social support by number of neurotic disorders

Perceived social support	No neurotic disorder	1 neurotic disorder	2+ neurotic disorders
	%	%	%
All adults			
No lack	57	47	66
Moderate lack	28	28	26
Severe lack	16	26	8
Base	*1348*	*209*	*8184*

Table 4.7 Proportion of adults with a neurotic disorder by perceived social support

	Perceived social support			
	No lack	Moderate lack	Severe lack	All *
	Percentage with neurotic disorder			
Women	17	21	41	20
Men	10	13	20	12
All adults	14	17	29	16
Bases				
*Women * *	*3356*	*1120*	*383*	*4908*
*Men * *	*2817*	*1431*	*524*	*4833*
*All adults * *	*6174*	*2550*	*907*	*9741*

* Bases for each level of social support do not sum to totals for all adults as data on social support are not available for some people (less than 1% overall)

Table 4.8 Presence of a neurotic disorder by perceived social support and stressful life events

Number of stressful life events	Perceived social support			
	No lack	Moderate lack	Severe lack	All
	Percentage with neurotic disorder			
0	9	10	18	10
1	14	17	29	17
2 or more	26	30	46	30
All adults	14	17	29	16
Bases				
0	*3020*	*1160*	*380*	*4620*
1	*1912*	*844*	*279*	*3036*
2 or more	*1182*	*546*	*247*	*1975*
All adults	*6174*	*2550*	*907*	*9741*

Table 4.9 Size of primary support group by family unit type and sex

Size of primary support group	Family unit type						
	Couple, no child(ren)	Couple & child(ren)	Lone parent & child(ren)	One person only	Adult with parents	Adult with one parent	All
	%	%	%	%	%	%	%
Women							
9 or more	65	60	41	56	58	40	58
4 - 8	31	35	46	37	36	50	36
0 - 3	5	5	14	8	7	10	6
Base	*1345*	*1942*	*494*	*592*	*419*	*115*	*4908*
Men							
9 or more	70	64	49	59	65	50	64
4 - 8	24	29	39	32	30	38	29
0 - 3	6	7	12	10	5	12	7
Base	*1236*	*1960*	*62*	*716*	*656*	*204*	*4833*
All adults							
9 or more	67	62	42	57	62	46	61
4 - 8	28	32	45	34	32	42	32
0 - 3	5	6	14	9	6	11	7
Base	*2581*	*3902*	*556*	*1308*	*1075*	*319*	*9741*

Table 4.10 Extent of social networks among those with and without a neurotic disorder

Type and size of social network	Any neurotic disorder	No neurotic disorder	All adults
	%	%	%
Household members that feel close to *			
0	5	2	2
1	53	58	57
2	15	18	18
3	7	9	9
4 or more	1	2	2
Lives alone	18	11	12
Relatives that don't live with, that feel close to: *			
0	12 ⎤	8 ⎤	8 ⎤
1	13 ⎬ 41	9 ⎬ 31	10 ⎬ 33
2	16 ⎦	15 ⎦	15 ⎦
3	13	12	12
4	11	12	12
5	8	8	8
6	7	9	8
7	3	4	4
8	3	5	4
9	2	2	2
10 or more	11	15	14
Don't know	1	1	1
Friends outside of household that feel close to: *			
0	9 ⎤	6 ⎤	6 ⎤
1	11 ⎬ 37	6 ⎬ 25	7 ⎬ 27
2	16 ⎦	12 ⎦	14 ⎦
3	12	11	12
4	11	13	12
5	9	8	8
6	11	14	13
7	2	2	2
8	4	4	4
9	1	1	1
10	6	8	8
11	0	0	0
12	3	5	4
13 or more	6	9	8
Don't know	0	0	0
Base	*1557*	*8184*	*9741*

* percentages within each group total 100%

Table 4.11 Size of primary support group by CIS-R score and sex

Primary support group	CIS-R score (grouped)						
	0-5	6-11	12-17	18+	0-11	12+	All
	%	%	%	%	%	%	%
Women							
9 or more	62	57	51	39	61	45	64
4 - 8	33	37	42	44	34	43	29
0 - 3	5	6	7	17	5	12	7
Base	*2917*	*1116*	*437*	*437*	*4034*	*874*	*4908*
Men							
9 or more	67	61	53	46	66	49	58
4 - 8	27	32	35	38	28	36	36
0 - 3	6	6	12	16	6	14	6
Base	*3539*	*773*	*265*	*256*	*4312*	*521*	*4833*
All adults							
9 or more	64	59	52	41	31	46	61
4 - 8	30	35	39	42	64	41	32
0 - 3	6	6	9	17	6	13	7
Base	*6456*	*1890*	*702*	*694*	*8346*	*1396*	*9741*

Table 4.12 Size of primary support group by neurotic disorder

Primary support group	Mixed anxiety and depressive disorder	Generalised Anxiety Disorder	Depressive episode	Phobia	Obsessive-Compulsive Disorder	Panic disorder	Any neurotic disorder	No neurotic disorder	All
	%	%	%	%	%	%	%	%	%
All adults									
9 or more	51	47	34	38	42	49	48	64	61
4 - 8	39	38	46	41	38	38	40	31	32
0 - 3	10	15	20	21	19	13	13	6	7
Base	*750*	*439*	*220*	*180*	*157*	*93*	*1557*	*8184*	*9741*

Table 4.13   Size of primary support group by number of neurotic disorders

Primary support group	No neurotic disorder	1 neurotic disorder	2+ neurotic disorders	All
	%	%	%	%
All adults				
9 or more	64	49	40	61
4 - 8	31	40	39	32
0 - 3	6	11	21	7
Base	*8184*	*1348*	*209*	*9741*

Table 4.14   Proportion of adults with a neurotic disorder by size of primary support group and sex

	Size of primary support group			
	9 +	4 - 8	0 - 3	All
	Percentage with neurotic disorder			
Women	15	24	36	20
Men	10	15	24	12
All adults	12	20	30	16
Bases				
Women	*2846*	*1745*	*318*	*4908*
Men	*3101*	*1387*	*345*	*4833*
All adults	*5947*	*3132*	*663*	*9741*

Table 4.15   Presence of a neurotic disorder by size of primary support group and stressful life events

Number of stressful life events	Size of primary support group			
	9 +	4 - 8	0 - 3	All
	Percentage with neurotic disorder			
0	7	13	18	10
1	13	21	33	17
2 or more	25	34	47	30
All adults	12	20	30	16
Bases				
0	*2890*	*1469*	*310*	*4669*
1	*1899*	*980*	*191*	*3070*
2 or more	*1158*	*683*	*162*	*2003*
All adults	*5947*	*3132*	*663*	*9741*

Table 4.16 Odds ratios of neurotic disorder and socio-demographic correlates of having a small primary support group (0 to 3 people)

		Adjusted O.R	95% C.I
Neurotic disorder	No neurotic disorder	1.00	....
	Neurotic disorder	2.10**	(1.74-2.52)
Sex	Men	1.00	....
	Women	0.76**	(0.63-0.92)
Ethnicity	White	1.00	
	West Indian/ African	1.35	(0.79-2.31)
	Asian/ Oriental	1.75**	(1.18-2.60)
	Other	2.27*	(1.14-4.51)
Family unit type	Couple, no children	1.00	....
	Couple & child(ren)	1.14	(0.91-1.42)
	Lone parent & child(ren)	2.10**	(1.52-2.89)
	One person only	1.42*	(1.08-1.86)
	Adult with parents	1.04	(0.75-1.44)
	Adult with one parent	1.82**	(1.22-2.72)
Qualifications	A level or higher	1.00	....
	GCSE/ O level	1.70**	(1.33-2.18)
	Other	1.61**	(1.18-2.20)
	None	2.26**	(1.78-2.87)
Employment status	Working full-time	1.00	....
	Working part-time	0.72**	(0.54-0.95)
	Unemployed	1.01	(0.77-1.33)
	Economically inactive	1.09	(0.88-1.34)
Occupation type	Non-manual	1.00	....
	Manual	1.21*	(1.01-1.45)
Tenure	Owner-occupier	1.00	....
	Renter	1.59**	(1.33-1.91)

Other factors included in the regression analysis, but found not to be independently associated with having a small primary support group were: long-standing physical illness, age, type of accommodation and locality

* p< 0.05, **p < 0.01

Table 4.17   Odds ratios of neurotic disorder, size of the primary support group, and socio-demographic correlates of perceiving a severe lack of social support

		Adjusted O.R	95% C.I
Neurotic disorder	No neurotic disorder	1.00	....
	Neurotic disorder	1.40**	(1.25-1.58)
Size of primary support group	9 or more	1.00	....
	4 to 8	3.52**	(2.94-4.21)
	0 to 3	1.80**	(1.64-1.98)
Sex	Men	1.00	....
	Women	0.59**	(0.53-0.65)
Age	16-24	1.00	....
	25-34	0.96	(0.82-1.13)
	35-44	0.88	(0.74-1.05)
	45-54	0.83*	(0.69-0.99)
	55-64	0.76**	(0.63-0.91)
Ethnicity	White	1.00	....
	West Indian/African	1.28	(0.91-1.83)
	Asian/Oriental	1.51**	(1.17-1.93)
	Other	1.17	(0.72-1.90)
Family unit type	Couple, no children	1.00	....
	Couple & child(ren)	1.03	(0.91-1.16)
	Lone parent & child(ren)	1.39**	(1.13-1.71)
	One person only	1.37**	(1.18-1.59)
	Adult with parents	1.39**	(1.15-1.69)
	Adult with one parent	1.92**	(1.47-2.49)
Qualifications	A level or higher	1.00	....
	GCSE/ O level	1.15*	(1.02-1.30)
	Other	1.22*	(1.05-1.43)
	None	1.29**	(1.14-1.47)
Employment status	Working full-time	1.00	....
	Working part-time	0.99	(0.87-1.14)
	Unemployed	1.24*	(1.06-1.46)
	Economically inactive	1.11	(0.98-1.25)
Occupation type	Non-manual	1.00	....
	Manual	1.19**	(1.08-1.31)

Other factors included in the regression analysis, but found not to be independently associated with perceiving a severe lack of social support were : long-standing physical illness, type of accommodation, tenure and locality.

* p< 0.05, **p < 0.01

Table 4.18 Participation in leisure activities

Activities	CIS-R scores (grouped)						
	0-5	6-11	12-17	18+	0-11	12+	All
	Percentage participating in each activity						
In and around the home							
TV/ radio	91	91	89	84	91	86	90
Reading books and newspapers	71	71	68	63	71	66	70
Listening to music	66	67	68	66	67	67	67
Entertaining friends or relatives	55	57	56	46	55	51	55
Gardening	48	41	41	32	46	37	45
Writing letters/ telephoning	35	39	42	32	36	37	36
Hobbies	33	36	38	31	34	34	34
Games	31	29	27	23	31	25	30
DIY/ car maintenance	30	21	20	17	28	19	27
Out of the home							
Visiting friends or relatives	76	76	77	68	76	72	75
Pubs, restaurants	70	69	62	57	70	60	69
Shopping	68	70	67	64	68	65	68
Going for a walk, walking the dog	55	51	52	46	54	49	53
Sports as a participant	51	45	39	31	50	35	48
Cinema, theatre, concerts	46	46	42	32	46	38	45
Library	21	23	21	20	21	21	21
Clubs, organisations	21	19	15	13	20	14	20
Sports as a spectator	22	16	15	11	20	13	19
Night clubs, discos	18	20	18	14	18	16	18
Church	15	15	14	10	15	12	15
Classes, lectures	10	10	8	8	10	8	10
Bingo, amusement arcades	7	7	7	8	7	7	7
Bookmakers, betting and gambling	5	4	4	5	5	4	5
Political activities	1	1	2	2	1	2	2
Base	*6456*	*1890*	*702*	*694*	*8346*	*1396*	*9741*

Table 4.19 Leisure activities by neurotic disorder

Leisure activities	Mixed anxiety and depressive disorder	Generalised Anxiety Disorder	Depressive episode	Phobia	Obsessive-Compulsive Disorder	Panic	Any neurotic disorder	No neurotic disorder
Percentage parcipating in each activity								
In and around the home								
TV/ radio	86	89	83	87	83	92	87	91
Reading books and newspapers	66	68	57	62	63	68	66	71
Listening to music	66	65	66	69	74	70	67	67
Entertaining friends or relatives	55	48	41	47	49	56	51	56
Gardening	39	37	27	22	33	42	37	46
Writing letters/ telephoning	40	32	28	41	37	41	38	36
Hobbies	37	32	24	33	34	43	35	34
Games	28	22	20	25	18	33	26	31
DIY/ car maintenance	19	20	13	13	14	20	19	28
Out of the home								
Visiting friends or relatives	75	70	65	71	71	78	73	76
Pubs, restaurants	62	59	56	52	61	68	61	70
Shopping	68	64	55	63	65	72	66	68
Going for a walk, walking the dog	52	49	46	40	43	54	49	54
Sports as a participant	38	31	27	34	26	33	36	50
Cinema, theatre, concerts	43	32	30	36	31	31	38	46
Library	21	20	20	18	16	22	21	21
Clubs, organisations	14	15	10	17	14	24	15	20
Sports as a spectator	14	13	13	12	10	16	14	20
Night clubs, discos	18	10	14	17	16	20	16	18
Church	12	14	11	11	11	15	13	15
Classes, lectures	9	7	9	9	8	9	9	10
Bingo, amusement arcades	7	5	6	10	10	13	7	7
Bookmakers, betting and gambling	4	6	5	3	5	7	4	5
Political activities	2	1	2	4	5	1	2	1
Base	*750*	*439*	*220*	*180*	*157*	*93*	*1557*	*8184*

Table 4.20 Number of leisure activities involved in by CIS-R score and sex

Number of leisure activities*	CIS-R score (grouped)						
	0-5	6-11	12-17	18+	0-11	12+	All
	%	%	%	%	%	%	%
Women							
10 or more	41	40	35	23	40	29	38
4 - 9	55	56	57	61	55	59	56
0 - 3	4	5	8	16	4	12	6
Base	*2917*	*1116*	*437*	*437*	*4034*	*874*	*4908*
Men							
10 or more	40	36	20	25	39	28	38
4 - 9	51	58	58	59	55	58	55
0 - 3	6	7	12	16	6	14	7
Base	*3539*	*773*	*265*	*256*	*4312*	*521*	*4833*
All adults							
10 or more	40	38	34	24	40	29	38
4 - 9	55	56	57	60	55	59	56
0 - 3	5	6	9	16	5	13	6
Base	*6456*	*1890*	*702*	*694*	*8346*	*1396*	*9741*

* the maximum possible number of activities was 26 (9 + 1 'other' in the home and 15 + 1 'other' out of the home).

Table 4.21 Number of leisure activities involved in by neurotic disorder

Number of leisure activities*	Mixed anxiety and depressive disorder	Generalised Anxiety Disorder	Depressive episode	Phobia	Obsessive-Compulsive Disorder	Panic	Any neurotic disorder	No neurotic disorder	All
	%	%	%	%	%	%	%	%	%
All adults									
10 or more	32	23	18	27	24	33	29	40	38
4 - 9	58	63	60	56	63	62	59	55	56
0 - 3	10	14	21	17	12	5	12	5	6
Base	*750*	*439*	*220*	*180*	*157*	*93*	*1557*	*8184*	*9741*

* the maximum possible number of activities was 26 (9 + 1 'other' in the home and 15 + 1 'other' out of the home).

Table 4.22 Number of leisure activities involved in by number of neurotic disorders

Number of leisure activities*	No neurotic disorder	1 neurotic disorder	2+ neurotic disorders	All
	%	%	%	%
All adults				
10 or more	40	30	18	38
4 - 9	55	58	64	56
0 - 3	5	11	18	6
Base	*1348*	*209*	*8184*	*9741*

* the maximum possible number of activities was 26
  (9 + 1 'other' in the home and 15 + 1 'other' out of the home).

Table 4.23 Proportion of adults with a neurotic disorder by number of leisure activities involved in

	Number of activities *			
	10 or more	4 - 9	0 - 3	All
	Percentage with neurotic disorder			
Women	15	21	41	20
Men	10	13	22	12
All adults	12	20	30	16
Bases				
Women	*1885*	*2751*	*272*	*4908*
Men	*1817*	*2676*	*341*	*4833*
All adults	*3702*	*5246*	*613*	*9741*

* the maximum possible number of activities was 26
  (9 + 1 'other' in the home and 15 + 1 'other' out of the home).

Table 4.24 Perceived social support by size of primary support group and sex

Perceived social support	Size of primary support group			
	9 +	4 - 8	0 - 3	All
	%	%	%	%
Women				
No lack	77	62	38	69
Moderate lack	19	28	36	23
Severe lack	4	11	27	8
Base	*2846*	*1745*	*318*	*4908*
Men				
No lack	65	50	37	59
Moderate lack	27	36	32	30
Severe lack	8	14	32	11
Base	*3101*	*1387*	*345*	*4833*
All adults				
No lack	71	57	29	64
Moderate lack	23	31	35	26
Severe lack	6	12	37	9
Base	*5947*	*3132*	*663*	*9741*

Table 4.25 Presence of a neurotic disorder by size of primary support group and perceived social support

Perceived social support	Size of primary support group			
	9 +	4 - 8	0-3	All
	Percentage with a neurotic disorder			
No lack	12	17	24	14
Moderate lack	12	20	27	17
Severe lack	21	30	41	29
All adults	12	20	30	16
Bases				
No lack	*2666*	*928*	*108*	*3702*
Moderate lack	*3062*	*1952*	*413*	*5246*
Severe lack	*219*	*253*	*142*	*613*
All adults	*5947*	*6132*	*663*	*9741*

Table 4.26 Number of leisure activities involved in by size of primary support group and sex

Number of leisure activities*	Size of primary support group			
	9 +	4 - 8	0 - 3	All
	%	%	%	%
Women				
10 or more	47	29	16	38
4 - 9	50	64	63	56
0 - 3	3	7	21	6
Base	*2846*	*1745*	*318*	*4908*
Men				
10 or more	43	30	17	38
4 - 9	52	60	62	55
0 - 3	4	10	22	7
Base	*3101*	*1387*	*345*	*4833*
All adults				
10 or more	45	30	16	38
4 - 9	52	62	62	56
0 - 3	4	8	21	6
Base	*5947*	*3132*	*663*	*9741*

* the maximum possible number of activities was 26
  (9 + 1 'other' in the home and 15 + 1 'other' out of the home).

Table 4.27 Presence of a neurotic disorder by size of primary support group and number of leisure activities involved in

Number of leisure activities*	Size of primary support group			
	9 +	4 - 8	0 - 3	All
	Percentage with neurotic disorder			
10 or more	10	17	19	12
4 – 9	14	19	30	20
0 – 3	22	35	35	30
All adults	12	20	30	16
Bases				
10 or more	*2666*	*928*	*108*	*3702*
4 – 9	*3062*	*1952*	*413*	*5246*
0 – 3	*219*	*253*	*142*	*613*
All adults	*5947*	*3132*	*663*	*9741*

* the maximum possible number of activities was 26
  (9 + 1 'other' in the home and 15 + 1 'other' out of the home).

Table 4.28 Number of leisure activities involved in by perceived social support and sex

Number of leisure activities*	Perceived social support			
	No lack	Moderate lack	Severe lack	All
	%	%	%	%
Women				
10 or more	43	33	20	39
4 - 9	53	62	66	56
0 - 3	4	6	14	6
Base	*3356*	*1120*	*383*	*4858*
Men				
10 or more	43	33	22	38
4 - 9	52	58	63	55
0 - 3	5	8	15	7
Base	*2817*	*1431*	*524*	*4772*
All adults				
10 or more	43	33	21	38
4 - 9	53	60	64	56
0 - 3	4	7	15	6
Base	*6174*	*2550*	*907*	*9741*

* the maximum possible number of activities was 26 (9 + 1 'other' in the home and 15 + 1 'other' out of the home).

Table 4.29 Presence of a neurotic disorder by perceived social support and number of leisure activities involved in

Number of leisure activities*	Perceived social support			
	No lack	Moderate lack	Severe lack	All
Percentage with neurotic disorder				
10 or more	10	15	23	12
4 - 9	16	16	27	20
0 - 3	23	30	48	30
All adults	14	17	29	16
Bases				
10 or more	*2645*	*843*	*190*	*5947*
4 - 9	*3250*	*1522*	*584*	*3132*
0 - 3	*279*	*185*	*132*	*663*
All adults	*6174*	*2550*	*907*	*9741*

* the maximum possible number of activities was 26 (9 + 1 'other' in the home and 15 + 1 'other' out of the home).

Table 4.30   Receipt of services by level of perceived social support

Adults with a neurotic disorder

Type of service	Perceived social support			
	No lack	Moderate lack	Severe lack	All
	Percentage of people receiving service			
Contact with a GP:				
in last 2 weeks, any reason	30	30	24	29
in last 12 months, physical complaint	80	77	74	78
in last 12 months, mental complaint	32	35	43	35
Professional counselling or therapy	7	10	13	9
Base	*849*	*442*	*263*	*1557*
Receipt of professional help if suffered stressful life event :				
Death of other relative	5	2	2	4
Base	*164*	*80*	*47*	*291*
Serious illness of close relative	16	13	16	15
Base	*158*	*82*	*53*	*293*
Seeking work unsuccessfully	19	29	23	23
Base	*117*	*70*	*62*	*250*
Serious problem with a close friend	26	22	20	23
Base	*143*	*105*	*72*	*319*
Valuable possessions lost/stolen	19	24	13	22
Base	*83*	*45*	*40*	*169*
Major financial crisis	21	26	20	22
Base	*84*	*58*	*34*	*175*
Break up of marriage/ relationship	12	19	20	16
Base	*77*	*40*	*34*	*150*

* Those not asked about counselling/therapy were assumed
to have no such treatment

Chapter 5   Use of alcohol, drugs and tobacco

This chapter looks at alcohol use, drug misuse, and cigarette smoking and their relation to neurotic disorder.

In this report, drug misuse includes the use of illegal drugs such as cannabis, stimulants and hallucinogens, and the extra-medical use of prescription medicines. The consumption of prescribed medication in general was covered in Report 2 of this series of reports on psychiatric morbidity[1].

5.1   Alcohol consumption

Obtaining information about people's drinking is difficult, and as a result, social surveys consistently record lower levels of alcohol consumption than would be expected from alcohol sales. This is due to a variety of reasons, such as underestimation of amounts drunk at home, poor recall and non-response bias[2].

The methodology used on this survey to categorise alcohol consumption is the same as that used by the General Household Survey (GHS)[3] and the 1993 Health Survey for England[4].

All survey informants, with the exception of proxy informants, were asked how often they had drunk each of the following five types of drink in the previous year and how much of each type they usually drank on any one day:

- Shandy (excluding bottles or cans which have very low alcohol content)
- Beer, lager, stout, cider
- Spirits or liqueurs
- Sherry or martini
- Wine

To enable comparison between people who consumed different types of drink, informants described their consumption in terms of standard measures which contained similar amounts of alcohol, one unit of alcohol being approximately equivalent to a half pint of beer, a single measure of spirits (1/6 gill), a glass of wine (about 4.5 fluid ounces) or a small glass of sherry or fortified wine (2 fluid ounces).

The alcohol consumption rating is calculated by multiplying the number of units of each type of drink consumed on a 'usual' day by a conversion factor relating to the frequency with which it was drunk, and totalling across all drinks:

Multiplying factors for converting drinking frequency and number of units consumed on a usual day into a number of units consumed per week.

Drinking frequency	Multiplying factor	
Almost every day	7.0	
5 or 6 times per week	5.5	
3 or 4 times per week	3.5	
Once or twice per week	1.5	
Once or twice per month	0.375	(1.5/4)
Once or twice per 6 months	0.058	(1.5/26)
Once or twice per year	0.029	(1.5/52)

This conversion method is somewhat rough and ready: it requires people to estimate the amounts drunk on a 'usual' day which for irregular drinkers is impossible to define. Also, the method does not take account of the wide variation in alcoholic strength of some drinks, particularly beers. Nevertheless it does enable the survey to identify broad groups according to alcohol consumption. Possible imprecisions in estimates are therefore relatively unimportant in this context.

Alcohol consumption categories, based on usual weekly consumption (units) over the previous 12 months

Abstainer in the past year	Informant drank no alcohol	
Occasional drinker	Under 1 unit per week	
	Men	**Women**
	(units per week)	
Light	1 - 10	1 - 7
Moderate	11 - 21	8 - 14

Over the recommended sensible level:

	Men	Women
Fairly heavy	22 - 35	15 - 25
Heavy	36 - 50	26 - 35
Very heavy	51 or more	36 or more

These alcohol consumption categories are used throughout the analyses, although in some tables categories may be combined for ease of interpretation and because of small base numbers. The term 'abstainers' includes people who drink alcohol but did not do so in the past 12 months. Adults who drank less than one unit per week are termed 'occasional drinkers' and those who drank at least one unit per week are termed 'regular drinkers'.

The category boundaries conform with the recommended sensible drinking levels for men and women, 21 units per week for men and 14 for women, and are compatible with those used in other OPCS surveys. Consumption above these levels is thought to be associated with increased health risks[5]. In each category the consumption levels for women are about 70% of those for men and are thought to be roughly equivalent in physiological terms. It is accepted, however, that the effects of alcohol are likely to vary between individuals and according to the circumstances in which alcohol is consumed.

Alcohol consumption by sex and age

Table 5.1 shows that one in five adults inter-

viewed for the survey abstained from drinking alcohol or drank only occasionally: 7% had not drunk alcohol in the past year and a further 12% drank less often than once a week.

Women were twice as likely as men to be abstainers or occasional drinkers (27% compared with 13%). In contrast, men were twice as likely as women to drink more than the recommended sensible level per week, 30% compared with 15%, and 8% of men and 2% of women drank very heavily. The data are consistent with the 1993 Health Survey for England for people aged 16 to 64. *(Table 5.1) (Figure 5.1)*

Compared with other adults, those aged 55 to 64 years were more likely to abstain or drink occasionally (32%) and less likely to drink more than the recommended sensible level (15%).*(Table 5.2)*

Alcohol consumption and neurosis

CIS-R score

Abstention and occasional drinking increased with CIS-R score, a general measure of neurotic psychopathology, from 19% among the lowest scorers to 30% among the highest scorers. Although drinking over the recommended sensible level hardly varied by CIS-R score, men with CIS-R scores of 12 or more were more likely to drink very heavily (11%) compared with those who scored less than 12 (7%). *(Table 5.3)*

Neurotic disorder

The relationship between alcohol consumption and having a neurotic disorder mirrors that found for those with a score of 12 or more on the CIS-R. Women with neurosis were more likely than those with no disorder to abstain or drink occasionally (33% compared with 25%), but the difference between men was barely significant (16% compared with 12%). However, men with neurosis were more likely than those with no disorder to drink very heavily (12% compared with 7%). *(Table 5.4)*

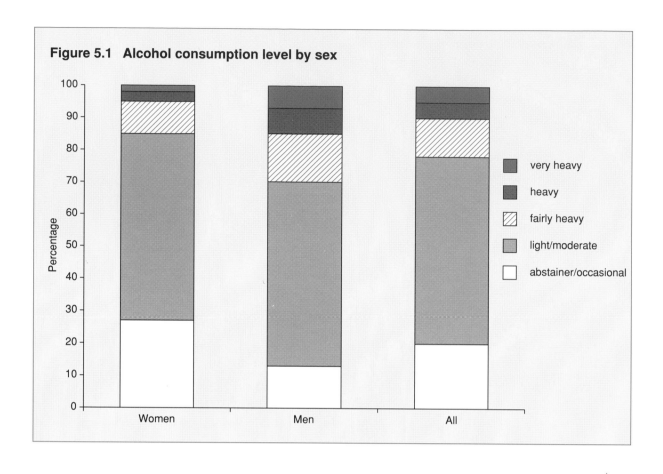

Figure 5.1 Alcohol consumption level by sex

Legend:
- very heavy
- heavy
- fairly heavy
- light/moderate
- abstainer/occasional

Compared with adults who had no neurotic disorder, those with phobia were much more likely to abstain or drink occasionally (40% compared with 19%) and this difference was particularly pronounced among women (48% compared with 25%). There were very few significant differences in alcohol consumption between men in relation to types of neurotic disorder. *(Table 5.5)*

Alcohol consumption was related to the number of neurotic disorders. Whereas 25% of women with no disorder abstained or drank occasionally, 32% of those with one disorder and 37% of those with comorbid disorders did so. Men with two or more disorders were more likely to be abstainers or drink occasionally (25%) than those with no disorder (12%). They were also more likely than those with no disorder to drink over the recommended sensible level (40% compared with 30%) as well as to drink very heavily (17% compared with 7%). *(Table 5.6)*

Odds ratios of factors associated with drinking very low and very high amounts

Two models were used to examine the independent association between having a neurotic disorder and various socio-demographic factors and (a) being an abstainer or occasional drinker, and (b) drinking very heavy amounts. The odds ratios produced show the increase or decrease in the odds of abstaining or drinking occasionally, or drinking very heavily that an individual with a particular characteristic had in relation to those in a reference group (for which the odds ratio is 1.00) while taking into account the possible confounding effects of other factors in the model.

Column (a) of Table 5.7 shows that, even after controlling for other factors, having a neurotic disorder was independently associated with increased odds of being an abstainer or occasional drinker in contrast with having no disorder (OR = 1.29). However, this association was relatively weak compared with those of other independent factors in the model.

The most striking factor associated with abstention or occasional drinking was ethnicity. Adults in non-White ethnic groups had greater odds of having this low level of consumption than White adults; odds were around 3 times greater for West Indians or Africans, and those in the 'other' category, and they were 14 times greater for Asian or Oriental adults. The model also confirmed earlier findings that sex and age were significantly associated with this level of alcohol consumption; men had far lower odds of abstention or drinking occasionally than women (OR = 0.41) and adults aged 16 to 54 had lower odds than those in the oldest age-group (ORs range from 0.31 to 0.66).

Model (b) showed that having a neurotic disorder was also independently associated with very heavy drinking (OR = 1.80). Again, a large association was found between ethnicity and drinking very heavily: compared with being White, being Asian or Oriental was associated with lower odds of drinking very heavily (OR = 0.30). Also, men had far greater odds of being heavy drinkers than women (OR = 3.26), and adults aged 16 to 54 years had greater odds than those in the oldest age-group (ORs were in the range: 1.74 to 2.25). *(Table 5.7)*

Prevalence of neurotic disorders by alcohol consumption

So far the discussion has looked at alcohol consumption among adults with a neurotic disorder. The focus now turns to examine how adults with varying levels of alcohol consumption differed in the extent to which they suffered a neurotic disorder.

Although adults with neurotic disorder made up 16% of the population, they comprised 24% of the population of abstainers and 22% of those drinking very heavily. Among women, 20% had a neurotic disorder which included 29% of abstainers and 30% of very heavy

drinkers. Thirteen percent of men had a neurotic disorder yet among those who drank only occasionally and those who drank very heavily, the proportions were 17% and 19% respectively. *(Table 5.8)*

Reasons for not drinking alcohol and neurotic disorder

All adults who said they did not drink alcohol nowadays were asked if they had always been non-drinkers or whether they used to drink but stopped. The majority, 58%, had never drunk alcohol and although neurotic adults appeared more likely to have drunk alcohol and given up than those without a disorder (59% compared with 40%), bases were very small and this difference was not statistically significant (table not shown). All non-drinkers were then asked the reason why they never drank or had stopped drinking from a pre-coded list. The two most commonly mentioned reasons by those who had never drunk alcohol were religious reasons and 'not liking it' whereas the predominant reason for stoping drinking was the concern for health. *(Table 5.9)*

5.2   Alcohol dependence

Three aspects of alcohol dependence were assessed for all informants who drank more than five units of alcohol in a single day at least once a week. These were loss of control, symptomatic behaviour and binge drinking.

Informants were classified as alcohol dependent if they responded positively to three or more of the following twelve statements:

Loss of control

1. Once I started drinking it was difficult for me to stop before I became completely drunk.

2. I sometimes kept on drinking after I had promised myself not to.

3. I deliberately tried to cut down or stop drinking, but I was unable to do so.
    continued

4. Sometimes I needed a drink so badly that I could not think of anything else.

Symptomatic behaviour

5. I have skipped a number of regular meals while drinking.

6. I have often had an alcoholic drink the first thing when I got up.

7. I have had a strong drink in the morning to get over the previous night's drinking.

8. I have woken up the next day not being able to remember some of the things I had done while drinking.

9. My hands shook a lot in the morning after drinking.

10. I need more alcohol than I used to, to get the same effect as before.

11. Sometimes I have woken up during the night or early morning sweating all over because of drinking.

Binge drinking

12. I have stayed drunk for several days at a time.

Adults were defined as having 'loss of control' or 'symptomatic behaviour' if they responded positively to 2 or more of the relevant statements and those who responded positively to the statement on binge drinking were defined as 'binge drinkers'. However, adults who satisfied the conditions for any one of these three components may not have met the criteria for being defined as alcohol dependent.

Eligible informants were given a self-completion questionnaire and asked to record whether a series of statements described their own experience in relation to drinking alcohol in the previous 12 months. These were the same as those used in the 1984 US Drinking Survey[7]. Adults who did not drink sufficiently large amounts of alcohol to be eligible for these questions were defined as non-dependent.

Alcohol dependence and consumption

Table 5.10 presents alcohol dependence among all adults according to their consumption level, including abstainers and occasional drinkers who were pre-defined as non-dependent. Overall, 8% of all men and 2% of all women were classified as alcohol dependent, and dependence increased at higher consumption levels, rising from 4% among moderate drinkers to 34% among the heaviest drinkers. This relationship was observed for men and women; men who drank moderate to heavy amounts were more likely than women to experience dependence.

The three aspects of alcohol dependence: symptomatic behaviour, loss of control, binge drinking - affected 3%, 2% and 1% of all adults respectively. These were increasingly prevalent at higher levels of alcohol consumption and were concentrated among those who drank over the recommended sensible level, and particularly among those who drank very heavily. Almost a quarter of very heavy drinkers exhibited symptomatic behaviour (23%), 16% experienced loss of control, and 9% experienced binge drinking. Rates of binge drinking among women did not rise dramatically with increased consumption, affecting just 3% of those who drank very heavily. For men however, binge drinking was particularly prevalent among very heavy drinkers (11%). *(Table 5.10)*

Alcohol dependence among regular drinkers

Focusing on adults who drank regularly, that is, those who drank at least one unit of alcohol per week can be regarded as being at risk of alcohol dependence. The overall rate of dependence was 3% for women and 9% for men. Dependence was most common among the youngest age group (13%) and least prevalent among the oldest age group (1%). A similar trend was found for men and women, and for the three areas of alcohol dependence. *(Table 5.11)*

Alcohol dependence and neurosis

CIS-R score

The proportion of regular drinkers affected by alcohol dependence increased with CIS-R score from 4% of those scoring under 6 to 16% of those scoring 18 or more. The same relationship was found for symptomatic behaviour and loss of control, and at a lower level, for binge drinking. (Table 5.12) (Figure 5.2)

Neurotic disorder

Regular drinkers with a neurotic disorder were more likely than those with no disorder to be alcohol dependent (12% compared with 5%) and similar relationships were found for symptomatic behaviour and loss of control. Binge drinking among regular drinkers, although negligible for women, was associated with neurotic disorder among men; 4% of men who drank regularly and had a neurotic disorder were binge drinkers compared with 1% of those with no such disorder. *(Table 5.13)*

Having more than one neurotic disorder was also associated with an increased likelihood of being alcohol dependent; while 5% of regular drinkers without a neurotic disorder were alcohol dependent, the proportions among those with one, and 2 or more disorders were 11% and 21% respectively. This relationship was also found for symptomatic behaviour and loss of control, and among men, for binge drinking. *(Table 5.14)*

Alcohol dependence, consumption and neurotic disorder

To demonstrate the magnitude of differences in alcohol dependence by neurotic disorder while controlling for consumption, regular drinkers were categorised into two broad groups: those who drank low to moderate amounts and those who drank over the recommended sensible level.

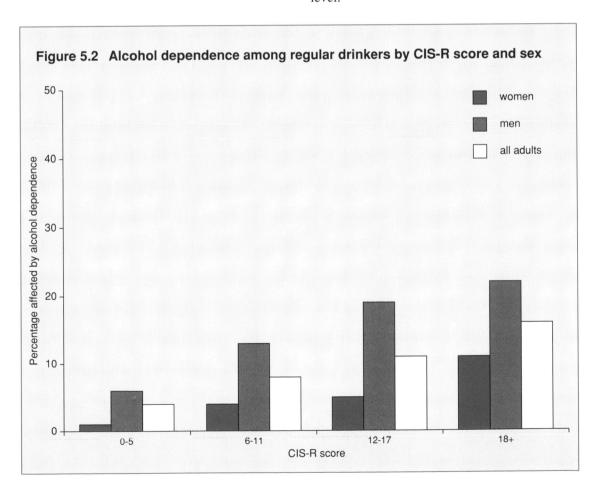

Figure 5.2 Alcohol dependence among regular drinkers by CIS-R score and sex

Looking at adults who drank more than the recommended sensible level, differences between those with neurosis and those without a neurotic disorder were pronounced: 28% of women and 41% of men who had a neurotic disorder were assessed as being alcohol dependent while the corresponding proportions among those without a neurotic disorder were 8% and 17%. Similar differences were found in symptomatic behaviour, loss of control, and among male regular-drinkers, in binge drinking. *(Table 5.15)*

Odds ratios of factors associated with alcohol dependence

Alcohol consumption had a major significant effect on dependence (ORs range from 6.77 among fairly heavy drinkers to 26.66 among very heavy drinkers), as did age with younger adults having greater odds of dependence than older ones (ORs range from 13.40 among adults aged 16 to 24 years to 2.73 among those aged 45 to 54 years). However, even after controlling for these and other significant factors, having a neurotic disorder was associated with a three-fold increase in the odds of dependence (OR = 3.02). This is comparable with the increase in odds of dependence associated with being male rather than female (OR = 3.33). *(Table 5.16)*

The prevalence of neurotic disorder by alcohol dependence

This section on alcohol dependence concludes by examining how the prevalence of neurotic disorder varies by alcohol dependence among regular drinkers. Whereas 14% of regular drinkers who were not alcohol dependent had a neurotic disorder, the proportion among dependent adults was 30%. *(Table 5.17)*

5.3 Alcohol problems

Any attempt to assess the proportion of people with problems associated with alcohol consumption is potentially controversial, because of the absence of agreed and widely accepted criteria defining alcohol-related problems. The survey covered a range of consequences of drinking too much: belligerence, social problems with a spouse, relatives or friends, health problems and problems with a job or the police[8].

Criteria for the definition of alcohol-related problems

Informants were classified as having had an alcohol problem if they answered 'yes' to any of the following statements.

Belligerence
I have got into a fight in a pub while drinking

or

I have got into a fight at home while drinking

or

I have got into a heated argument while drinking

Spouse problems
Spouse asked subject to drink less or act differently when drinking

Relative problems
A relative asked subject to drink less or act differently when drinking

Friend problems
A friend (including girlfriend/boyfriend, a co-resident, or anyone else) asked subject to drink less or act differently when drinking

or subject agrees with the statement:

My drinking has interfered with my spare time activities or hobbies

Job problems
I have lost a job or nearly lost one because of drinking

Police problems
I had trouble with the police about drinking when driving was not involved

or

I have been arrested for driving after drinking

or

A police office questioned me or warned me because of my drinking

continued

Health problems

I had an illness connected with drinking which kept me form working or doing my regular activities for a week or more

or

A doctor suggested that I cut down on my drinking

or

I felt that my drinking was becoming a serious threat to my physical health

Accidents

My drinking contributed to getting involved in an accident in which someone was hurt or property, such as a car, was damaged

or

My drinking contributed to my getting hurt in an accident in a car or elsewhere.

All adults who drank 5 or more units of alcohol on a single day per week were given a self completion questionnaire which asked them to record whether they had experienced any one of 16 alcohol-related problems in the previous 12 months. Those who did not consume sufficiently large amounts of alcohol to be eligible for these questions were defined as not having an alcohol problem.

Alcohol problems and consumption

Individuals vary greatly in their susceptibility to the effects of drink, and the amount of alcohol that is likely to result in impairment must also vary from individual to individual. Nevertheless, the increase in alcohol-related problems with consumption is very clear.

Twelve percent of all adults had experienced an alcohol-related problem, predominantly belligerence (8%). Three percent had health problems and 6% had a social problem. Although only 2% of adults who drank lightly had alcohol problems, the proportion rose to 13% of moderate drinkers and 63% among very heavy drinkers.

Problems were more common among men (19%) than women (5%). Nevertheless, belligerence was still the most widely experienced problem. The disparity between the proportions of men and women with alcohol problems remained even after controlling for consumption level. For example, among those who drank fairly heavily, 16% of women and 37% of men had experienced a problem. Among adults who drank very heavily, 54% of women and 66% of men had an alcohol-related problem. Belligerence however was almost equally common among men and women who were heavy drinkers (around 28%) and among very heavy drinkers (43%). *(Table 5.18)*

Alcohol problems and neurosis

Among regular drinkers, that is those who can be regarded as being at risk of having alcohol problems, 15% had an alcohol problem, with men being 3 times more likely to have had a problem than women (22% compared with 7%). *(Table 5.19)*

CIS-R score

Among regular drinkers, the proportion suffering an alcohol problem increased from 13% among those scoring under 6 on the CIS-R to 24% among the highest scorers (18 or more). *(Table 5.19)*

Neurotic disorder

Regular drinkers with a neurotic disorder were more likely to have had an alcohol problem (22%) than those with no such disorder (14%). A similar pattern was found for belligerence, health problems, problems with a spouse, relative or friend, and for problems with the police, and accidents. Since alcohol problems were relatively rare among adults who drank below the recommended sensible level, there was little variation in alcohol problems between adults with and without a neurotic disorder in this group. *(Table 5.20)*

Alcohol problems increased with the number of neurotic disorders. There was a two-fold

89

increase in the proportion of men and women with alcohol problems from those with no disorder to those with 2 or more disorders (6% to 13% for women and 20% to 41% for men). *(Table 5.21)*

Odds ratios of factors associated with alcohol problems

Table 5.22 shows the odds of regular drinkers having an alcohol problem, after controlling for neurotic disorder, alcohol consumption, and various socio-demographic characteristics using multiple logistic regression analysis. The analysis confirms that there was a significant independent association between neurosis and alcohol problems; having a neurotic disorder was associated with a two-fold increase in the odds of having an alcohol problem (OR = 1.93).

As expected, the level of alcohol consumption was the most important factor (ORs ranging from 6.93 to 23.88 according to consumption level compared with drinking low to moderate amounts). Other factors which had an independent association with alcohol problems included age (ORs range from 3.96 to 1.41 with increasing age, compared with being age 55 to 64), sex (OR associated with being male = 3.00). One factor which decreased the odds of having alcohol problems was ethnicity; being Asian or Oriental, or being West Indian or African was associated with far lower odds than being White (ORs = 0.26 and 0.34). *(Table 5.22)*

Prevalence of neurotic disorder among adults with alcohol problems

Overall 21% of regular drinkers with an alcohol problem had a neurotic disorder in contrast with 14% of regular drinkers with no alcohol problem. Those who had problems with their health, their relationship with friends, or with accidents were the most likely to have a neurotic disorder (around 32%). *(Table 5.23)*

Alcohol problems and alcohol dependence

As expected, an association between alcohol-related problems and dependence was clearly evident: 85% of regular drinkers who were alcohol dependent had an alcohol problem compared with 10% of their non-dependent counterparts. The existence of a neurotic disorder had little effect on this relationship. *(Table 5.24)*

5.4 Drug use

All informants with the exception of those interviewed by proxy were asked about their use of drugs including sedatives, tranquillisers, cannabis, amphetamines, cocaine, heroin, opiates, hallucinogens, Ecstasy and glue. In the case of prescribed drugs, most usually sedatives and tranquillisers, we were only interested in their extra-medical use. Hence, information in this chapter is not comparable with that presented in Chapter 2 of Report 2 on the medical use of drugs.

Extra-medical and illicit use was ascertained by presenting informants with a list of drugs and asking if they had used any of these without a prescription, more than was prescribed for them, or to get high. Sedatives and tranquillisers were placed highest on the list to deter adults who did not use illicit drugs but did misuse medication from assuming the questions did not apply to them.

List of commonly used drugs

Sleeping pills, Barbiturates, Sedatives, Downers, Seconal

Tranquillisers, Valium, Lithium

Cannabis, Marijuana, Hash, Dope, Grass, Ganja, Kif

Amphetamines, Speed, Uppers, Stimulants, Qat

Cocaine, Coke, Crack

Heroin, Smack

continued

Opiates other than heroin: Demerol, Morphine, Methadone, Darvon, Opium, DF118

Psychedelics, Hallucinogens: LSD, Mescaline, Acid, Peyote, Psilocybin (magic) mushrooms

Ecstasy

Solvents, Inhalants, Glue, Amyl nitrate

Drug categories used in analysis

Sleeping tablets Tranquillisers	Hypnotics
Cannabis	Cannabis
Amphetamines Cocaine/crack	Stimulants
Hallucinogens/psychedelics Ecstasy	Hallucinogens including Ecstasy
Heroin Opiates Solvents, inhalants	Others

The questions on drug use and the drug categories were drawn from the drugs section of the Diagnostic Interview Schedule (DIS)[9] and were used in the U.S. ECA study[10]. Questions on injecting drugs and needle sharing were added.

Informants who reported using any of the drugs listed either without a prescription, or at more than the prescribed dosage, or to get high, were then asked if they had taken the drug more than five times in their life. Those who had done so and had also taken the drug in the past twelve months formed the population of interest.

Informants may have exaggerated or under-reported their drug use according to how acceptable they perceived their drug taking to be, both to people around them and also to the interviewer. Despite assurances of confidentiality and using a self-completion questionnaire, some informants may still have had concerns over confidentiality and been reluctant to report their drug use truthfully. Therefore, results presented here may be an underestimate of actual drug use, but they do provide estimates of an absolute minimum.

The type of drugs taken are generally presented in broad groupings owing to the small numbers of people who had taken some types. Informants can appear in several categories if they took more than one type of drug. For some analyses it has only been possible to categorise drug takers into three groups: those who only took cannabis, those who only took other drugs, and those who took both cannabis and other drugs.

Use of drugs

One in twenty people had taken at least one of the drugs listed in the questionnaire in the past year. Drug use was less common among women than men (4% compared with 7%). Cannabis was the most commonly used drug (5%) followed by stimulants (1%) and hallucinogens (1%). Men were more likely to use cannabis (6%) than women (3%) and although the use of hallucinogens, including Ecstasy, was negligible among women, 2% of men had taken them in the past year. *(Table 5.25)*

These estimates compare very well with the self-reported use of drugs during 1991 estimated by the 1992 British Crime Survey (BCS)[11] which interviewed 7,000 people aged 12 to 59 years about their knowledge and use of drugs. There were no significant differences in the estimates of drug use between the two surveys although the BCS population was somewhat younger.

Use of drugs was far more common among the youngest age-group and declined rapidly with age; whereas 15% of adults aged 16 to 24 had used a drug in the past year, the proportion among 25 to 34 year olds was 6% and fell to 1% in the oldest age-group. This trend was found for the use of cannabis, stimulants and hallucinogens but not for hypnotics and other drugs. The use of cannabis, stimulants and hallucinogens was highest among men in the youngest age-group (18%, 6% and 7% respectively). *(Table 5.26)*

Among adults who had taken drugs in the past year, nine out of ten had used cannabis (89%), one in five had taken stimulants or hallucinogens (20% and 18%) and one in eight had taken hypnotic drugs (12%). Men were more likely to take every of type of drug than women except hypnotics; 21% of women who took drugs, took hypnotics compared with 6% of men. *(Table 5.27)*

About a third (30%) of adults who used cannabis also took non-cannabinoid drugs, primarily stimulants or hallucinogens. Cannabis was used by almost all those who took stimulants or hallucinogens and over a third of adults who had taken hypnotics. *(Table 5.28)*

In summary, 63% of drug takers only used cannabis and a further 11% took cannabis as well as other drugs. The remaining quarter (26%) only took non-cannabinoid drugs, the majority of whom were only taking hypnotics (67%). In contrast, only 15% of adults who took both cannabis and other drugs, had taken hypnotics (table not shown).

Drug use and neurosis

CIS-R score

Overall, rates of drug use increased with CIS-R score. The use of cannabis alone and of non-cannabinoid drugs was twice as common among adults who scored 12 or more than those with lower scores. Among men, drug use reached its peak among those scoring 18 or more on the CIS-R (9%), whereas for women the proportion of drug-takers with CIS-R scores of 12 or above was 15%. *(Table 5.29)*

Neurotic disorder

Adults with neurotic disorder were more than twice as likely to have used a drug in the past year than others (10% compared with 4%).

Consumption of drugs was particularly high among adults who suffered from phobia (16%), panic (15%) and depression (14%). *(Table 5.30)*

In addition to the presence of a neurotic disorder, drug use was associated with the number of neurotic disorders. Overall, 15% of those with two or more disorders had used any drug in the past year, as had 9% of those with just one disorder and 4% of those with none.

Among those with neurosis, there was no significant difference in the proportions who only took cannabis by the number of disorders. However, marked differences were found in the use of *any* non-cannabinoid drug, rising from 1% of adults with no neurotic disorder to 4% of those with one disorder, and 10% of those with two or more disorders. Differences were most marked among adults who *only* took non-cannabinoid drugs. *(Table 5.31)*

Odds ratios of factors associated with drug use

Having a neurotic disorder was found to be independently associated with increased odds of using drugs (OR = 2.66) even after various socio-demographic characteristics were controlled for, using multiple logistic regression analysis. Alcohol consumption was also considered in the model.

Several other factors, however, had a greater association with the odds of using drugs than having a neurotic disorder. The most notable of these was age. Younger adults had far greater odds of using drugs compared with adults in the oldest age-group (OR = 13.48 for 16 to 24 year olds and 7.05 for 25 to 34 year olds). Secondly, alcohol consumption was highly associated with drug use: adults who drank over the recommended sensible level had much higher odds of drug use than those who abstained or drank occasionally (ORs range from 3.95 to 4.80). *(Table 5.32)*

Prevalence of neurotic disorder by drug use

So far we have discussed how adults varied in their use of drugs in relation to whether they suffered a neurotic disorder. This section now concentrates on those adults who took drugs and whether they suffered a neurotic disorder.

Neurotic disorder was twice as common among adults who used drugs (31%) than among those who did not (15%). The prevalence of neurosis was highest (45%) among those who only took non-cannabinoid drugs (two-thirds of whom only took hypnotics) and lowest among those who only took cannabis (28%). *(Table 5.33)*

Method of drug use and neurotic disorder

Four percent of all drug users who had taken drugs in the past year had injected them (that is, 0.2% of all adults aged 16 to 64). This represented 8% of drug takers who had a neurotic disorder and 2% of those with no disorder, but these estimates are based on just 20 adults and differences between them are not significant (table not shown). Of all those who had injected, 18 responded to the question about needle sharing: 5 said they had shared a needle in the previous month, and 13 said they had not shared.

5.5 Drug dependence and problems

All adults who had taken drugs and had taken them in the past year were asked questions about their experiences relating to aspects of dependence and problems caused by drug use. As for drug use, the questions were based on the drugs section of the DIS which were used in the ECA study in the US. Informants who gave positive responses to any of the relevant questions were classified as drug-dependent or having a drug-related problem. Dependency could also be categorised according to the type of drug causing it. A self-completion questionnaire was used for privacy.

Definition of drug dependence and problems
A pre-requisite is that the drug(s) must have been taken either:

- without a prescription
- more than was prescribed for the subject
- or to get high

and that they were taken in the past year, having been taken more than 5 times in the subject's life.

Drug dependence
The informant was defined as drug dependent if any of the following experiences applied to her/him in the past 12 months:

1. used any one of these drugs every day for two weeks or more

2. used any one of these drugs to the extent that she/he felt she/he needed it or was dependent on it

3. tried to cut down on any drugs but felt she/he couldn't do it

4. needed larger amounts of the drug(s) to get an effect, or that she/he could no longer get high on the amounts she/he used to use

5. had withdrawal symptoms such as feeling sick because she/he stopped or cut down on any of these drugs.

Drug problems
The informant was defined as having a drug problem if any of the following experiences applied to her/him in the past 12 months:

1. had a health problem such as fits, an accidental overdose, a persistent cough, or an infection as a result of using any of these drugs

2. drugs caused her/him considerable problems with family or friends, at work or at school or with the police

3. had emotional or psychological problems from taking drugs, such as feeling crazy or paranoid, or depressed or uninterested in things

4. talked to a doctor about any problems she/he may have had from taking drugs

5. talked to any other professional about any problems she/he may have had from taking drugs

6. had any drug problem which interfered with her/his life or activities a lot.

Overall 41% of drug takers were drug dependent and 25% had a drug-related problem. The higher proportion of drug takers with dependence than with problems reflects the less stringent criteria for assessing dependence than problems. *(Table 5.34)*

Drug takers aged 25 to 34 years were the least likely to have been drug dependent (28%) compared with those in other age-groups (47%). Later in this section, these age differences are shown to persist after controlling for the types of drugs used, that is, whether cannabis or non-cannabinoid drugs were used alone, or whether they were used in combination, as well as socio-demographic characteristics (see Table 5.37) . This suggests that drug takers aged 25 to 34 may have been using drugs in greater moderation than other drug takers.

Drug related problems decreased with age from 34% among the youngest adults (aged 16 to 24) to 11% among older adults but, once other factors were taken into account using multiple logistic regression, age was not a significant factor associated with drug problems (see Table 5.38).

Drug dependence and problems, and neurosis

Drug takers with a neurotic disorder were more likely to suffer from dependence (60%) as well as to have a drug-related problem (36%) compared with their counterparts who did not have a disorder, of whom 32% were dependent and 20% had a problem. *(Table 5.35)*

Drug dependence, neurosis and the type of drug taken

All adults who responded positively to any of the statements about drug dependence were asked to state the type of drug that caused this. Over half the adults who took hypnotics were dependent on them (53%) and over a third of

cannabis takers were dependent on it. Similarly, 22% of stimulant takers, 13% of hallucinogen takers and 30% of those who took other drugs were dependent on those drugs (table not shown).

Adults who had only taken cannabis in the past year were far less likely to be dependent on it (24%) than those who had taken any other drugs as well (63%). In contrast, dependence on non-cannabinoid drugs was more prevalent among adults who took only non-cannabinoid drugs (57%) than those who took cannabis as well. Also, the prevalence of neurosis and drug dependence was particularly high among adults who only took non-cannabinoid drugs (34%). These findings are largely due to the high proportion of adults who only took hypnotics (67%) among those who only took only non-cannabinoid drugs. *(Table 5.36)*

Odds ratios of factors associated with drug dependence and drug problems

The association between neurotic disorder and the type of drug used , and the odds of either being dependent or having problems, were explored using multiple logistic regression modelling which also controlled for alcohol use and various socio-demographic characteristics. The models were based on all adults who had taken drugs and their drug use was categorised according to whether they solely took cannabis (the reference group), or solely used non-cannabinoid drugs, or if they used both cannabis and other drugs.

Having a neurotic disorder greatly increased the odds of being drug dependent (OR = 3.41) even after controlling for the types of drugs used and other factors. It is also noteworthy that compared with only taking cannabis, taking only non-cannabinoid drugs was associated with increased odds of being drug dependent (OR = 4.37) and an even greater increase was associated with taking cannabis combined with non-cannabinoid drugs (OR = 9.55). This confirms the earlier findings on drug dependence by the type of drugs taken.

Having broadly controlled for the types of drugs taken, it is interesting that the youngest drug takers did not have significantly different odds of drug dependency compared with those aged 35 to 64, but 25 to 34 year old drug takers were less likely to suffer dependence (OR = 0.37). Ethnicity was another important factor associated with drug dependence although it was not significantly associated with drug use; West Indian or African adults had higher odds of being drug dependent than White adults (OR = 9.06). *(Table 5.37)*

The odds of having a drug problem were also associated with neurotic disorder and the type of drugs used. Adults with a neurotic disorder had around twice the odds of having a drug problem (OR = 2.02) as those with no disorder. Compared with adults who solely took cannabis, odds were again greater among those who took cannabis in combination with other drugs (OR = 10.11) than for those who solely took other drugs (OR = 2.01). *(Table 5.38)*

Sex, age and neurotic disorder by drug dependence and problems

How did drug takers who experienced dependency or problems differ from those who did not, in relation to sex, age and the number of neurotic disorders? For this comparison, data are also presented for adults who did not take drugs and for the whole population.

Drug takers were more likely to be male (65%) than female (35%) but this did not vary significantly by whether adults were affected by drug dependence or problems. This confirms the earlier findings that whereas women were less likely to take drugs, those who did take drugs were as likely as men to experience dependency and problems.

Over half (54%) of all drug takers were aged 16 to 24 years and adults who were drug dependent were more likely to be in this age-group (62%) than those who were not depend-

ent (49%). In contrast, drug-takers who suffered dependency were less likely to be aged 25 to 34 (21%) compared with those who were not dependent (37%).

Similarly, 16 to 24 year olds were over-represented among drug takers who experienced problems (73%) compared with those who did not (47%), and drug takers aged 25 to 34, and 35 to 44 were under-represented.

Neurotic disorders were more prevalent among drug takers who had experienced dependency or problems than among those who had not experienced them. The prevalence of neurosis among dependent drug takers was 46% and among their non-dependent counterparts, it was 21%. Among drug takers who had drug-related problems, 45% had a neurotic disorder compared with 27% of those who did not have a drug problem.*(Table 5.39)*

5.6 Cigarette smoking

All informants, except proxies, were asked if they had ever smoked cigarettes, and if they smoked nowadays. This did not include cigar and pipe smoking. If they did smoke, they were asked how many cigarettes they smoked a day. This was prompted firstly for weekdays, and then for weekends to get a more accurate average daily consumption. Adults were grouped into categories, depending on whether they had ever smoked, and the average daily amount smoked. These questions were asked in the 1992 General Household Survey (GHS) and the 1993 Health Survey for England.

Cigarette smoking categories

Never regularly smoked	
Ex-smokers	
Current smokers:	
Light	Less than 10 a day
Moderate	Less than 20 a day, but more than 10
Heavy	More than 20 a day

The GHS found that consumption of cigarettes is under-estimated by 10% in comparison with Customs and Excise data on the number of cigarettes released into the UK. This is partly due to adults understating their consumption of cigarettes, either deliberately or by mistake, and to a lesser extent, denying that they smoke altogether. Other factors include non-response bias and non-coverage of the whole population as adults not living in private households and those under 16 years of age are excluded from the GHS.

This survey found that almost a third of all adults (32%) smoked cigarettes; 8% were light smokers, 13% were moderate and 11% were heavy smokers. These proportions did not differ between men and women but although the proportions of non-smokers was roughly equal, men were more likely than women to be ex-smokers (25% compared with 18%). These data compare very well with the 1993 Health Survey for adults aged 16 to 64 years. *(Table 5.40)*

Although the youngest adults were the most likely to smoke (37%) and smoking decreased with age, younger adults were the lightest smokers; 14% were light smokers compared with 8% overall. Heavy smoking was more common among adults aged between 25 and 54 years. This age relationship was found for men and women. *(Table 5.41)*

Cigarette smoking and neurosis

CIS-R score

Cigarette smoking increased with informants' overall scores on the CIS-R, rising from 28% among the lowest scorers (0 to 5) to 48% among those scoring 18 or more. High CIS-R scores were also associated with heavier smoking; although the proportion of light smokers remained fairly constant with increasing CIS-R score, moderate smoking increased slightly and heavy smoking increased significantly (from 9% among the lowest scorers to 23% among the highest). *(Figure 5.3)*

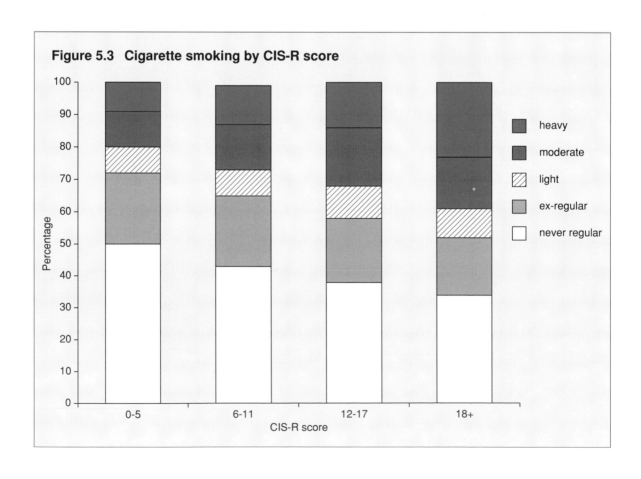

Figure 5.3 Cigarette smoking by CIS-R score

Differences in the amount smoked between men and women were generally very small and non-significant at each level of CIS-R score. One exception to this is that men who scored 12 to 17 on the CIS-R were more likely to smoke than women (50% compared with 38%). *(Table 5.42)*

Neurotic disorder

Adults with a neurotic disorder were more likely than other adults to smoke, and smoke more heavily. Whereas 44% of adults with neurosis smoked, only 29% of other adults did so. The corresponding proportions for moderate smoking were 17% and 12%, and for heavy smoking, 18% and 10%.

Adults with depressive disorder or panic disorder were the most likely to smoke (56% and 55%) in contrast with 44% of all adults with neurosis. They were also the most likely to be heavy smokers (26% compared with 18% of all adults with neurosis). *(Table 5.43)*

Both smoking and heavy smoking increased with the number of neurotic disorders. Twenty-nine per cent of adults with no disorder smoked and 10% did so heavily, the corresponding proportions among those with one disorder were 43% and 17%, and among those with two or more disorders, 54% and 26%. Differences were found for men and women, but owing to small bases, differences between those with one disorder and those with 2 or more disorders, were not statistically significant. *(Table 5.44)*

Odds ratios of factors associated with cigarette smoking

Even after controlling for alcohol consumption, drug use and various socio-demographic factors using multiple logistic regression modelling, neurotic disorder was identified as a significant independent factor associated with cigarette smoking. With reference to adults with no neurotic disorder, those with a neurotic disorder had 1.60 times greater odds of smok-

ing cigarettes. However, the use of drugs was the factor most strongly associated with smoking. Not surprisingly, cannabis users had far greater odds of being smokers than those who did not take cannabis, but odds were higher for those who used cannabis in combination with other drugs (OR = 10.30) than for those who used cannabis alone (OR = 5.42). Also, higher levels of alcohol consumption were associated with increased odds of being a smoker compared with being an abstainer or occasional drinker (ORs range from 1.28 to 2.98). Once again, ethnicity was an important factor; both Asian or Oriental , and West Indian or African adults had lower odds of smoking cigarettes than their White counterparts (ORs = 0.33 and 0.47). *(Table 5.45)*

Prevalence of neurotic disorder by cigarette smoking

Having looked at how cigarette smoking varies in relation to neurotic disorder, the focus turns to what proportion of smokers and non-smokers had a neurotic disorder. Those who had never smoked were the least likely to suffer a disorder (12%), followed by the ex-smokers (15%); the most likely to do so were the heavy smokers (26%). Differences between those who had never smoked and those who had stopped smoking were relatively small, but for men ex-smokers were more likely to suffer from neurosis than those who had never smoked (12% compared with 8%). *(Table 5.46)*

5.7 Alcohol consumption, use of drugs and cigarette smoking

Use of alcohol, drugs and tobacco were found to be significantly and independently associated with the odds of having a neurotic disorder and of these, drug use was the most highly associated. Compared with not taking any drugs, the greatest increase in the odds of having neurosis was associated with taking drugs other than cannabis (which in two-thirds of cases, meant only taking hypnotics) (OR = 3.46), followed by taking such drugs in combination with cannabis

(OR = 2.46). Taking cannabis only was associated with around twice the odds of being neurotic (OR = 1.92). Being a heavy smoker was also associated with higher odds of having neurosis (OR = 1.36). The odds of having a neurotic disorder for adults who drank heavily or very heavily were similar to those of the reference group of adults who abstained or drank only occasionally (OR = 1.04). However, for adults who drank low to moderate amounts, the odds of having neurosis were lower than for those who abstained or drank occasionally (OR = 0.71) as were the odds for those who drank fairly heavily (OR = 0.63). *(Table 5.50)*

References

1 Meltzer, H., Gill, B., Petticrew, M. and Hinds, K., (1995). *The OPCS Surveys of Psychiatric Morbidity in Great Britain, Report 2*, HMSO London

2 Goddard, E., (1991). *Drinking in England and Wales in the late 1980s.* HMSO London, Chapter 1

3 Thomas, M., Goddard, E., Hickman, M., and Hunter, P.,(1994). *1992 General Household Survey.* HMSO London

4 Bennett, N., Dodd, T., Flatley, J., Freeth, S., and Bolling, K., (1995) *Health Survey for England 1993*. HMSO London

5 *Alcohol and the heart in perspective: sensible limits reaffirmed.* Report of a joint working group of the Royal College of Physicians, the Royal College of Psychiatrists and the Royal College of General Practitioners. June 1995

6 Goddard, E, *op cit,* Chapter 9

7 Hilton, M.E., (1991) A note on measuring drinking problems in the 1984 National Alcohol Survey in (eds) Clark and Hilton, *Alcohol in America,* State University of New York: Albany

8 Ibid

9 Robins, L. N., Helzer, J.E., Croughan, J. and Ratcliff, K.S., (1981). National Institute of Mental Health Diagnostic Interview Schedule: Its History, Characteristics, and Validity, *Archives of General Psychiatry,* vol 38, pp 381-389.

10 *Psychiatric Disorders in America, The Epidemiologic Catchment Area Study*, edited by Robins, L.N., and Reiger, D.A., (1991) Free Press New York

11 Mott, J., and Mirlees-Black, C., *Self-Reported Drug Misuse in England and Wales: findings from the 1992 British Crime Survey: Research and Planning Unit Paper 89* (1995) Home Office London, Table B4.2

Table 5.1 Alcohol consumption level by sex: a comparison with the 1993 Health Survey

Alcohol consumption level (number of units per week)	Psychiatric Morbidity Survey		Health Survey Adults aged 16-64	
	%		%	
Women				
Abstainer*	9	27	9	27
Occasional drinker (under 1)	17		18	
Light (1-7)	41		41	
Moderate (over 7-14)	17		17	
Fairly heavy (over 14-25)	10		10	
Heavy (over 25-35)	3	15	3	15
Very heavy (over 35)	2		3	
Base	*4882*		*6947*	
Men				
Abstainer*	5	13	6	12
Occasional drinker (under 1)	8		7	
Light (1-10)	34		33	
Moderate (over 10-21)	23		22	
Fairly heavy (over 21-35)	15		16	
Heavy (over 35-50)	8	30	9	32
Very heavy (over 50)	8		7	
Base	*4810*		*6313*	
All adults				
Abstainer*	7	20	8	20
Occasional drinker	12		12	
Light	38		37	
Moderate	20		20	
Fairly heavy	12		13	
Heavy	5	22	6	23
Very heavy	5		5	
Base **	*9692*		*13260*	

Source: 1993 Health Survey for England data, OPCS

*   Includes informants who had not had an alcoholic drink in the past twelve months

**   Bases exclude 49 informants for whom alcohol consumption could not be measured on the Psychiatric Morbidity Survey

Table 5.2   Alcohol consumption level by age (grouped) and sex

Alcohol consumption level	Age (grouped)					
	16-24	25-34	35-44	45-54	55-64	All
Women						
Abstainer	9 ⎤ 21	7 ⎤ 22	8 ⎤ 24	9 ⎤ 28	16 ⎤ 43	9 ⎤ 26
Occasional drinker	12 ⎦	15 ⎦	16 ⎦	20 ⎦	27 ⎦	17 ⎦
Light	40	46	41	40	37	41
Moderate	21	18	19	18	11	17
Fairly heavy	11 ⎤	9 ⎤	11 ⎤	10 ⎤	7 ⎤	10 ⎤
Heavy	3 ⎥ 18	3 ⎥ 15	3 ⎥ 16	2 ⎥ 14	1 ⎥ 9	3 ⎥ 15
Very heavy	4 ⎦	2 ⎦	2 ⎦	1 ⎦	1 ⎦	2 ⎦
Base	*912*	*1216*	*1055*	*928*	*771*	*4882*
Men						
Abstainer	7 ⎤ 15	4 ⎤ 9	4 ⎤ 7	5 ⎤ 12	8 ⎤ 20	5 ⎤ 13
Occasional drinker	8 ⎦	5 ⎦	7 ⎦	7 ⎦	12 ⎦	8 ⎦
Light	33	32	34	37	38	34
Moderate	22	23	25	21	21	23
Fairly heavy	15 ⎤	17 ⎤	14 ⎤	15 ⎤	11 ⎤	15 ⎤
Heavy	5 ⎥ 29	10 ⎥ 35	8 ⎥ 30	8 ⎥ 30	6 ⎥ 21	8 ⎥ 30
Very heavy	10 ⎦	8 ⎦	8 ⎦	8 ⎦	4 ⎦	8 ⎦
Base	*943*	*1213*	*995*	*911*	*748*	*4810*
All adults						
Abstainer	8 ⎤ 18	6 ⎤ 16	6 ⎤ 18	7 ⎤ 20	12 ⎤ 32	7 ⎤ 20
Occasional drinker	10 ⎦	10 ⎦	12 ⎦	14 ⎦	20 ⎦	12 ⎦
Light	37	39	37	38	38	38
Moderate	21	20	22	19	16	20
Fairly heavy	13 ⎤	13 ⎤	13 ⎤	12 ⎤	9 ⎤	12 ⎤
Heavy	4 ⎥ 24	6 ⎥ 25	6 ⎥ 23	5 ⎥ 22	3 ⎥ 15	5 ⎥ 22
Very heavy	7 ⎦	5 ⎦	5 ⎦	5 ⎦	2 ⎦	5 ⎦
Base	*1856*	*2428*	*2050*	*1839*	*1518*	*9692*

Table 5.3 Alcohol consumption level by CIS-R score (grouped) and sex

Alcohol consumption level	CIS-R score (grouped)						
	0 - 5	6 - 11	12 - 17	18+	0 - 11	12+	All
	%	%	%	%	%	%	%
Women							
Abstainer	8 ⎤ 26	8 ⎤ 25	12 ⎤ 30	16 ⎤ 35	8 ⎤ 26	14 ⎤ 32	9 ⎤ 27
Occasional drinker	17 ⎦	17 ⎦	18 ⎦	19 ⎦	17 ⎦	18 ⎦	17 ⎦
Light	43	40	39	33	42	36	41
Moderate	18	18	16	16	18	16	17
Fairly heavy	10 ⎤	11 ⎤	6 ⎤	10 ⎤	10 ⎤	8 ⎤	10 ⎤
Heavy	2 ⎥ 14	3 ⎥ 17	4 ⎥ 15	3 ⎥ 16	2 ⎥ 15	4 ⎥ 15	3 ⎥ 15
Very heavy	2 ⎦	2 ⎦	4 ⎦	3 ⎦	2 ⎦	4 ⎦	2 ⎦
Base	*2903*	*1111*	*434*	*434*	*4014*	*868*	*4882*
Men							
Abstainer	6 ⎤ 13	3 ⎤ 10	7 ⎤ 13	7 ⎤ 22	5 ⎤ 12	7 ⎤ 18	5 ⎤ 13
Occasional drinker	7 ⎦	6 ⎦	7 ⎦	15 ⎦	7 ⎦	11 ⎦	8 ⎦
Light	35	37	31	30	35	30	34
Moderate	23	22	23	18	23	20	23
Fairly heavy	15 ⎤	14 ⎤	13 ⎤	14 ⎤	15 ⎤	13 ⎤	15 ⎤
Heavy	8 ⎥ 29	9 ⎥ 32	9 ⎥ 33	5 ⎥ 30	8 ⎥ 30	7 ⎥ 32	8 ⎥ 30
Very heavy	7 ⎦	9 ⎦	11 ⎦	12 ⎦	7 ⎦	11 ⎦	8 ⎦
Base	*3523*	*770*	*263*	*254*	*4293*	*517*	*4810*
All							
Abstainer	7 ⎤ 19	6 ⎤ 19	10 ⎤ 24	13 ⎤ 30	7 ⎤ 19	11 ⎤ 27	7 ⎤ 20
Occasional drinker	12 ⎦	12 ⎦	14 ⎦	18 ⎦	12 ⎦	16 ⎦	12 ⎦
Light	38	39	36	32	38	34	38
Moderate	21	20	18	16	20	17	20
Fairly heavy	13 ⎤	12 ⎤	9 ⎤	11 ⎤	13 ⎤	10 ⎤	12 ⎤
Heavy	5 ⎥ 22	6 ⎥ 23	6 ⎥ 22	4 ⎥ 21	5 ⎥ 22	5 ⎥ 22	5 ⎥ 22
Very heavy	4 ⎦	5 ⎦	7 ⎦	6 ⎦	5 ⎦	6 ⎦	5 ⎦
Base	*6426*	*1881'*	*698*	*688*	*8306*	*1386*	*9692*

Table 5.4 Alcohol consumption level by neurotic disorder and sex

Alcohol consumption level	Women			Men			All adults		
	Neurotic disorder	No neurotic disorder	All	Neurotic disorder	No neurotic disorder	All	Neurotic disorder	No neurotic disorder	All
	%	%	%	%	%	%	%	%	%
Abstainer	14 ⎤ 33	8 ⎤ 25	9 ⎤ 27	6 ⎤ 16	5 ⎤ 12	5 ⎤ 13	11 ⎤ 26	7 ⎤ 19	7 ⎤ 20
Occasional drinker	19 ⎦	17 ⎦	17 ⎦	10 ⎦	7 ⎦	8 ⎦	16 ⎦	12 ⎦	12 ⎦
Light	36	42	41	31	35	34	34	39	38
Moderate	16	18	17	20	23	23	17	20	20
Fairly heavy	8 ⎤	10 ⎤	10 ⎤	14 ⎤	15 ⎤	15 ⎤	10 ⎤	13 ⎤	12 ⎤
Heavy	3 ⎬ 15	2 ⎬ 15	3 ⎬ 15	8 ⎬ 33	8 ⎬ 30	8 ⎬ 30	5 ⎬ 22	5 ⎬ 22	5 ⎬ 22
Very heavy	3 ⎦	2 ⎦	2 ⎦	12 ⎦	7 ⎦	8 ⎦	7 ⎦	5 ⎦	5 ⎦
Base	*952*	*3929*	*4882*	*594*	*4217*	*4810*	*1546*	*8146*	*9692*

Table 5.5 Alcohol consumption level by type of neurotic disorder and sex

Alcohol consumption level	Neurotic disorder								
	Mixed anxiety and depressive disorder	Generalised Anxiety Disorder	Depressive episode	All phobias	Obsessive-Compulsive Disorder	Panic disorder	Any neurotic disorder	No neurotic disorder	All
	%	%	%	%	%	%	%	%	%
Women									
Abstainer	11	17	18	26	17	13	14	8	9
Occasional drinker	19	17	16	23	17	20	19	17	17
(Abstainer + Occasional)	*30*	*34*	*34*	*48*	*34*	*33*	*33*	*25*	*27*
Light	40	34	34	31	36	33	36	42	41
Moderate	15	18	17	9	11	14	16	18	17
Fairly heavy	7	9	6	8	12	12	8	10	10
Heavy	4	2	4	3	3	5	3	2	3
Very heavy	4	3	5	1	3	3	3	2	2
(Fairly heavy + Heavy + Very heavy)	*15*	*14*	*15*	*12*	*18*	*21*	*15*	*15*	*15*
Base	482	247	131	121	100	50	952	3929	4882
Men									
Abstainer	5	8	11	11	8	2	6	5	5
Occasional drinker	11	12	8	10	10	6	10	7	8
(Abstainer + Occasional)	*16*	*20*	*20*	*21*	*18*	*8*	*16*	*12*	*13*
Light	31	27	30	25	24	43	31	35	34
Moderate	22	16	16	23	18	9	20	23	23
Fairly heavy	12	15	14	16	23	14	14	15	15
Heavy	8	7	8	4	4	6	8	8	8
Very heavy	11	14	12	12	12	20	12	7	8
(Fairly heavy + Heavy + Very heavy)	*31*	*36*	*35*	*31*	*39*	*40*	*33*	*30*	*30*
Base	263	187	87	57	57	43	594	4217	4810
All adults									
Abstainer	9	13	15	21	14	8	11	7	7
Occasional drinker	16	15	13	19	15	13	16	12	12
(Abstainer + Occasional)	*25*	*28*	*28*	*40*	*28*	*21*	*26*	*19*	*20*
Light	37	31	32	29	32	38	34	39	38
Moderate	18	18	16	14	14	12	17	20	20
Fairly heavy	9	11	9	10	16	13	10	13	12
Heavy	5	4	5	3	4	6	5	5	5
Very heavy	7	8	8	4	6	11	7	5	5
(Fairly heavy + Heavy + Very heavy)	*21*	*24*	*23*	*18*	*26*	*30*	*22*	*22*	*22*
Base	745	434	218	178	157	93	1546	8146	9692

Table 5.6   Alcohol consumption level by number of neurotic disorders and sex

Alcohol consumption level	Women			Men			All adults		
	None	One	Two or more	None	One	Two or more	None	One	Two or more
	%	%	%	%	%	%	%	%	%
Abstainer	8 ⎤ 25	13 ⎤ 32	20 ⎤ 37	5 ⎤ 12	5 ⎤ 15	13 ⎤ 25	7 ⎤ 19	10 ⎤ 26	17 ⎤ 32
Occasional drinker	17 ⎦	19 ⎦	17 ⎦	7 ⎦	10 ⎦	12 ⎦	12 ⎦	16 ⎦	15 ⎦
Light	42	37	34	35	32	23	39	35	30
Moderate	18	16	14	23	21	12	20	18	13
Fairly heavy	10 ⎤	8 ⎤	8 ⎤	15 ⎤	13 ⎤	18 ⎤	13 ⎤	10 ⎤	12 ⎤
Heavy	2 ⎬ 15	3 ⎬ 15	3 ⎬ 15	8 ⎬ 30	8 ⎬ 32	5 ⎬ 40	5 ⎬ 22	5 ⎬ 22	4 ⎬ 24
Very heavy	2 ⎦	4 ⎦	3 ⎦	7 ⎦	11 ⎦	17 ⎦	5 ⎦	6 ⎦	8 ⎦
Base	*3929*	*824*	*128*	*4217*	*515*	*78*	*8146*	*1339*	*207*

Table 5.7   Significant odds ratios associated with alcohol consumption (a) of less than one unit per week and (b) of more than 35 units (women) or 50 units (men) per week

		(a) Less than one unit per week		(b) more than 35/50 units per week	
		Adjusted O.R	95% C.I	Adjusted O.R	95% C.I
Neurotic disorder	No neurotic disorder	1.00	....	1.00	....
	Neurotic disorder	1.29**	(1.12-1.49)	1.80**	(1.42-2.28)
Sex	Male	0.41**	(0.36-0.47)	3.26**	(2.56-4.16)
	Female	1.00	....	1.00	....
Age	16-24	0.31**	(0.24-0.39)	2.25**	(1.46-3.48)
	25-34	0.40**	(0.33-0.49)	1.93**	(1.30-2.87)
	35-44	0.49**	(0.40-0.60)	2.13**	(1.41-3.22)
	45-54	0.66**	(0.55-0.79)	1.74**	(1.15-2.62)
	55-64	1.00	....	1.00	....
Ethnicity	White	1.00	....	1.00	....
	West Indian or African	2.98**	(2.07-4.28)	0.62	(0.25-1.53)
	Asian or Oriental	14.23**	(10.79-18.77)	0.30*	(0.11-0.80)
	Other	3.18**	(1.92-5.27)	0.21	(0.03-1.42)
Qualifications	A level or higher	1.00	....		
	GCSE/O level	1.43**	(1.23-1.70)		
	Other qualifications	1.55**	(1.27-1.89)		
	No qualifications	1.70**	(1.44-2.00)		
Family unit type	Couple, no children	1.00	....	1.00	....
	Couple & child(ren)	1.17 *	(1.00-1.36)	0.65**	(0.50-0.86)
	Lone parent & child(ren)	1.13	(0.89-1.44)	0.79	(0.43-1.42)
	One person	0.94	(0.78-1.15)	1.68**	(1.26-2.25)
	Adult with parents	1.96**	(1.51-2.55)	0.99	(0.67-1.46)
	Adult with one parent	1.35	(0.94-1.94)	1.32	(0.82-2.10)
Employment status	Working full-time	1.00	....	1.00	....
	Working part-time	1.07	(0.91-1.26)	0.77	(0.55-1.07)
	Unemployed	1.55**	(1.27-1.91)	0.61**	(0.44-0.84)
	Economically inactive	1.99**	(1.73-2.30)	0.41**	(0.29-0.58)
Occupation type	Non-manual	1.00	....	1.00	....
	Manual	1.28**	(1.13-1.44)	1.63**	(1.33-2.00)
Tenure	Owner/occupier	1.00	....	1.00	....
	Renter	1.35**	(1.19-1.54)	1.45**	(1.17-1.80)

Significance: *   p<0.05   ** p<0.01

Factors entered in model (a) which were not significantly associated with the level of alcohol consumption were: accommodation and locality and for model (b) were: qualifications, accommodation and locality

Table 5.8   Prevalence of neurotic disorder by alcohol consumption level and sex

Neurotic disorder	Alcohol consumption level							
	Abstainer	Occasional drinker	Light	Moderate	Fairly heavy	Heavy	Very heavy	All
Women	%	%	%	%	%	%	%	%
Neurotic disorder	29	21	17	18	16	26	30	20
No neurotic disorder	71	79	83	82	84	74	70	80
Base	*461*	*844*	*2010*	*848*	*485*	*127*	*107*	*4882*
Men	%	%	%	%	%	%	%	%
Neurotic disorder	14	17	11	11	12	12	19	12
No neurotic disorder	86	83	89	89	88	88	81	88
Base	*258*	*362*	*1661*	*1085*	*704*	*368*	*373*	*4810*
All adults	%	%	%	%	%	%	%	%
Neurotic disorder	24	20	14	14	14	16	22	16
No neurotic disorder	76	80	86	86	86	84	78	84
Base	*718*	*1206*	*3671*	*1933*	*1189*	*495*	*480*	*9692*

Table 5.9   Reasons for not drinking alcohol by whether subject has always been a non - drinker or has stopped drinking and neurotic disorder

Base:Adults who did not drink alcohol

Reason why a non - drinker/ stopped drinking	Never drank alcohol			Stopped drinking alcohol		
	Neurotic disorder	No neurotic disorder	All	Neurotic disorder	No neurotic disorder	All
	Percentage of adults who gave each reason*					
Religious reasons	34	41	40	1	10	7
Does not like it	46	43	44	17	22	21
Parental advice	16	6	8	2	1	1
Health reasons	4	8	7	49	46	47
Cannot afford it	1	3	3	13	8	9
Other reason	22	14	15	31	28	29
Base	*86*	*326*	*411*	*82*	*219*	*301*

* Percentages add to more than 100 as informants may have reported more than one reason

Table 5.10   Alcohol dependence by alcohol consumption level and sex

Alcohol dependence	Alcohol consumption level						
	Abstainer/ Occasional drinker	Light	Moderate	Fairly heavy	Heavy	Very heavy	All
Women		*Percentage affected by dependence*					
Alcohol dependence	-	0	2	6	23	29	2
Symptomatic behaviour	-	0	1	3	12	19	1
Loss of control	-	0	1	3	10	17	1
Binge drinking	-	-	-	0	5	3	0
Base	*1305*	*2010*	*848*	*485*	*127*	*107*	*4882*
Men							
Alcohol dependence	-	1	6	13	18	36	8
Symptomatic behaviour	-	0	2	6	9	24	4
Loss of control	-	0	2	7	8	15	3
Binge drinking	-	0	1	2	1	11	1
Base	*620*	*1661*	*1085*	*704*	*368*	*373*	*4810*
All adults							
Alcohol dependence	-	1	4	10	20	34	5
Symptomatic behaviour	-	0	2	5	10	23	3
Loss of control	-	0	1	5	8	16	2
Binge drinking	-	0	0	1	2	9	1
Base	*1924*	*3671*	*1933*	*1189*	*495*	*480*	*9692*

Base excludes 49 informants for whom alcohol consumption could not be measured

Table 5.11   Alcohol dependence by age (grouped) and sex

Base: Regular drinkers

Alcohol dependence	Age					
	16-24	25-34	35-44	45-54	55-64	All
	Percentage affected by dependence					
Women						
Alcohol dependence	8	3	2	1	0	3
Symptomatic behaviour	5	2	0	1	0	2
Loss of control	3	1	1	1	0	2
Binge drinking	1	0	-	0	-	0
Base	*722*	*950*	*802*	*663*	*440*	*3576*
Men						
Alcohol dependence	19	11	6	4	2	9
Symptomatic behaviour	11	6	3	2	1	5
Loss of control	7	5	3	2	1	4
Binge drinking	4	2	1	0	0	2
Base	*802*	*1100*	*889*	*802*	*598*	*4191*
All adults						
Alcohol dependence	13	8	4	3	1	6
Symptomatic behaviour	8	4	2	2	1	3
Loss of control	5	3	2	2	1	3
Binge drinking	2	1	1	0	0	1
Base	*1523*	*2050*	*1691*	*1466*	*1038*	*7767*

Table 5.12   Alcohol dependence by CIS-R score (grouped) and sex

Base: Regular drinkers

Alcohol dependence	CIS-R score (grouped)							
	0 - 5	6 - 11	12 - 17	18+	0 - 11	12+	All	
	Percentage affected by alcohol dependence							
Women								
Alcohol dependence	1	4	5	11	2	8	3	
Symptomatic behaviour	1	2	5	6	1	6	2	
Loss of control	1	1	3	8	1	5	2	
Binge drinking	0	0	1	1	0	1	0	
Base	*2157*	*834*	*303*	*282*	*2991*	*586*	*3576*	
Men								
Alcohol dependence	6	13	19	22	8	20	9	
Symptomatic behaviour	3	8	11	11	4	11	5	
Loss of control	3	6	6	15	3	10	4	
Binge drinking	1	2	4	5	1	4	2	
Base	*3067*	*696*	*229*	*198*	*3764*	*427*	*4191*	
All								
Alcohol dependence	4	8	11	16	5	13	6	
Symptomatic behaviour	2	5	7	8	3	8	3	
Loss of control	2	3	4	11	2	7	3	
Binge drinking	1	1	2	3	1	2	1	
Base	*5224*	*1530*	*532*	*481*	*6754*	*1013*	*7767*	

Table 5.13   Alcohol dependence by neurotic disorder and sex

Base: Regular drinkers

Alcohol dependence	Women			Men			All adults		
	Neurotic disorder	No neurotic disorder	All women	Neurotic disorder	No neurotic disorder	All men	Neurotic disorder	No neurotic disorder	All adults
	Percentage affected by dependence								
Alcohol dependence	7	2	3	19	8	9	12	5	6
Symptomatic behaviour	5	1	2	10	4	5	7	3	3
Loss of control	5	1	2	10	3	4	7	2	3
Binge drinking	1	0	0	4	1	2	2	1	1
Base	*639*	*2937*	*3576*	*496*	*3694*	*4191*	*1136*	*6632*	*7767*

109

Table 5.14 Alcohol dependence by the number of neurotic disorders and sex

Base: Regular drinkers

Alcohol dependence	Women			Men			All adults		
	None	One	Two or more	None	One	Two or more	None	One	Two or more
Percentage affected by dependence									
Alcohol dependence	2	7	12	8	17	34	5	11	21
Symptomatic behaviour	1	4	9	4	9	19	3	7	13
Loss of control	1	4	12	3	8	23	2	6	17
Binge drinking	0	1	2	1	3	10	1	2	5
Base	*2937*	*558*	*81*	*3694*	*438*	*59*	*6632*	*996*	*139*

Table 5.15 Alcohol dependence by neurotic disorder, alcohol consumption level and sex

Base: Regular drinkers

Alcohol dependence	Neurotic disorder			No neurotic disorder			All		
	Alcohol consumption level			Alcohol consumption level			Alcohol consumption level		
	Low to moderate	Over recom- mended sensible level	All	Low to moderate	Over recom- mended sensible level	All	Low to moderate	Over recom- mended sensible level	All
Percentage affected by dependence									
Women									
Alcohol dependence	1	28	7	1	8	2	1	12	3
Symptomatic behaviour	1	19	5	0	4	1	0	7	2
Loss of control	1	18	5	0	4	1	0	6	2
Binge drinking	-	4	1	-	1	0	-	1	0
Base	*495*	*144*	*639*	*2363*	*575*	*2937*	*2858*	*719*	*3576*
Men									
Alcohol dependence	5	41	19	2	17	8	3	20	9
Symptomatic behaviour	1	25	10	1	10	4	1	12	5
Loss of control	2	20	10	1	7	3	1	9	4
Binge drinking	1	8	4	0	3	1	0	4	2
Base	*299*	*197*	*496*	*2446*	*1248*	*3694*	*2746*	*1445*	*4191*
All adults									
Alcohol dependence	3	35	12	2	14	5	2	18	6
Symptomatic behaviour	1	22	7	1	8	3	1	10	3
Loss of control	1	20	7	1	6	2	1	8	3
Binge drinking	0	7	2	0	2	1	0	3	1
Base	*794*	*341*	*1136*	*4809*	*1822*	*6632*	*5603*	*2164*	*7767*

Table 5.16   Significant odds ratios associated with being alcohol dependent (compared with not being dependent)

Base: Regular drinkers

		Adjusted OR	95% confidence interval
Alcohol consumption level	Light/ moderate	1.00	....
	Fairly heavy	6.77**	(5.03-9.11)
	Heavy	15.20**	(10.95-21.10)
	Very heavy	26.66**	(19.60-36.27)
Neurotic disorder	No neurotic disorder	1.00	....
	Neurotic disorder	3.02**	(2.34-3.89)
Sex	Male	3.33**	(2.51-4.40)
	Female	1.00	....
Age	16-24	13.40**	(6.81-26.37)
	25-34	6.94**	(3.60-13.39)
	35-44	3.88**	(1.95-7.74)
	45-54	2.73**	(1.35-5.52)
	55-64	1.00	....
Ethnicity	White	1.00	....
	West Indian/African	0.64	(0.21-1.90)
	Asian/Oriental	0.17	(0.02-1.25)
	Other	2.68	(0.96-7.46)
Family unit type	Couple, no children	1.00	....
	Couple & child(ren)	1.00	(0.71-1.40)
	Lone parent & child(ren)	1.92 *	(1.08-3.41)
	One person	1.60**	(1.13-2.28)
	Adult with parents	1.44	(0.95-2.19)
	Adult with one parent	1.60	(0.95-2.67)
Employment status	Working full-time	1.00	....
	Working part-time	2.19**	(1.53-3.11)
	Unemployed	1.18	(0.84-1.65)
	Economically inactive	1.56 *	(1.10-2.22)
Accommodation type	Detached	1.00	....
	Semi-detached	0.92	(0.64-1.30)
	Terraced	1.39	(0.99-1.96)
	Flat or maisonette	1.55 *	(1.05-2.30)

Significance: * $p<0.05$ ** $p<0.01$

Factors entered in the model which were not significantly associated with alcohol dependence were: qualifications, occupation type, tenure and locality

111

Table 5.17   Prevalence of neurotic disorder by alcohol dependence and sex

Base: Regular drinkers

	Alcohol dependence	Symptomatic behaviour	Loss of control	Binge drinking	No alcohol dependence	All
	%	%	%	%	%	%
Women						
Neurotic disorder	44	52	57	[6]	17	18
No neurotic disorder	56	48	43	[4]	83	82
Base	*107*	*63*	*53*	*9*	*3469*	*3576*
Men						
Neurotic disorder	26	26	30	30	10	12
No neurotic disorder	74	74	70	70	90	88
Base	*371*	*199*	*161*	*66*	*3819*	*4191*
All adults						
Neurotic disorder	30	32	36	34	14	15
No neurotic disorder	70	68	64	66	86	85
Base	*479*	*262*	*214*	*75*	*7289*	*7767*

Table 5.18 Alcohol problems by consumption level and sex

Base: all adults

Alcohol problem	Abstainer/ Occasional drinker	Light	Moderate	Fairly heavy	Heavy	Very heavy	All
	Percentage with each alcohol problem						
Women							
Belligerence	-	1	8	12	27	43	4
Health problems	-	0	1	2	8	18	1
Problems with friends	-	0	1	4	11	11	1
Problems with spouse	-	0	1	1	7	15	1
Problems with relatives	-	0	1	3	8	10	1
Police problems	-	0	0	1	2	2	0
Accidents	-	-	0	0	3	3	0
Job problems	-	-	-	-	-	-	-
Any alcohol problem	**-**	**1**	**9**	**16**	**35**	**54**	**5**
Base	*1305*	*2010*	*848*	*485*	*127*	*107*	*4882*
Men							
Belligerence	-	2	11	27	29	43	13
Health problems	-	0	3	8	16	28	5
Problems with friends	-	1	4	9	10	22	5
Problems with spouse	-	1	2	9	12	17	4
Problems with relatives	-	1	2	4	4	19	3
Police problems	-	1	3	5	6	14	3
Accidents	-	0	1	3	3	9	2
Job problems	-	-	-	1	2	2	0
Any alcohol problem	**-**	**3**	**17**	**37**	**46**	**66**	**19**
Base	*620*	*1661*	*1085*	*704*	*368*	*373*	*4810*
All adults							
Belligerence	-	1	10	21	29	43	8
Health problems	-	0	2	6	14	26	3
Problems with friends	-	0	3	7	10	19	3
Problems with spouse	-	0	2	6	11	16	2
Problems with relatives	-	0	1	3	5	17	2
Police problems	-	0	2	3	5	12	2
Accidents	-	0	1	2	3	8	1
Job problems	-	-	0	2	2	0	0
Any alcohol problem	**-**	**2**	**13**	**29**	**43**	**63**	**12**
Base	*1924*	*3671*	*1933*	*1189*	*495*	*480*	*9692*

Table 5.19   Alcohol problems by CIS-R score (grouped) and sex

Base: Regular drinkers

Alcohol problems	CIS-R score (grouped)						
	0-5	6-11	12-17	18+	0-11	12+	All
	Percentage with alcohol problems						
Women							
Belligerence	4	8	6	14	5	10	6
Health problems	0	2	3	6	1	4	1
Problems with friends	1	1	2	7	1	4	1
Problems with spouse	0	1	2	4	1	3	1
Problems with relatives	1	1	2	3	1	3	1
Police problems	0	1	0	1	0	1	0
Accidents	0	0	1	1	0	1	0
Job problems	-	-	-	-	-	-	-
Any alcohol problem	**5**	**10**	**10**	**17**	**6**	**13**	**7**
Base	*2157*	*834*	*303*	*282*	*2991*	*586*	*3576*
Men							
Belligerence	12	19	20	24	14	22	14
Health problems	4	8	12	18	5	14	6
Problems with friends	4	8	10	14	5	12	6
Problems with spouse	4	7	8	12	4	10	5
Problems with relatives	3	6	3	8	3	5	3
Police problems	3	6	7	8	3	7	4
Accidents	1	2	6	4	2	5	2
Job problems	0	1	1	3	0	2	1
Any alcohol problem	**19**	**27**	**32**	**33**	**20**	**33**	**22**
Base	*3067*	*696*	*229*	*198*	*3764*	*427*	*4191*
All adults							
Belligerence	9	13	12	18	10	15	11
Health problems	3	5	7	11	3	9	4
Problems with friends	3	4	6	10	3	8	4
Problems with spouse	2	4	5	8	3	6	3
Problems with relatives	2	3	3	5	2	4	2
Police problems	2	3	3	4	2	4	2
Accidents	1	1	3	2	1	3	1
Job problems	0	0	0	1	0	1	0
Any alcohol problem	**13**	**18**	**20**	**24**	**14**	**22**	**15**
Base	*5224*	*1530*	*532*	*481*	*6754*	*1013*	*7767*

Table 5.20   Alcohol problems by neurotic disorder, consumption level and sex

Base: Regular drinkers

Alcohol problem	Neurotic disorder			No neurotic disorder			All adults		
	Alcohol consumption level			Alcohol consumption level:			Alcohol consumption level:		
	Light to moderate	Over recom- mended sensible level	All	Light to moderate	Over recom- mended sensible level	All	Light to moderate	Over recom- mended sensible level	All
Percentage with each alcohol problem									
Women									
Belligerence	4	27	10	2	17	5	3	19	6
Health problems	1	16	4	0	3	1	0	5	1
Problems with friends	0	18	4	0	3	1	0	6	1
Problems with spouse	0	13	3	0	2	1	0	4	1
Problems with relatives	1	8	2	0	4	1	0	5	1
Police problems	0	3	1	0	1	0	0	2	0
Accidents	0	2	1	-	1	0	0	1	0
Job problems	-	-	-	-	-	-	-	-	-
Any alcohol problem	**5**	**40**	**13**	**3**	**21**	**6**	**3**	**25**	**7**
Base	*495*	*144*	*639*	*2363*	*575*	*2937*	*2858*	*719*	*3576*
Men									
Belligerence	7	43	21	5	30	14	5	32	14
Health problems	2	32	14	1	12	5	1	15	6
Problems with friends	3	26	12	2	10	5	2	12	6
Problems with spouse	1	24	10	1	10	4	1	12	5
Problems with relatives	1	14	6	1	7	3	1	8	3
Police problems	2	18	8	1	6	3	2	8	4
Accidents	2	11	5	0	4	2	1	4	2
Job problems	-	4	2	-	1	0	-	1	1
Any alcohol problem	**12**	**65**	**33**	**8**	**44**	**20**	**8**	**47**	**22**
Base	*299*	*197*	*496*	*2446*	*1248*	*3694*	*2746*	*1445*	*4191*
All adults									
Belligerence	5	36	14	4	26	10	4	27	11
Health problems	1	25	8	1	9	3	1	12	4
Problems with friends	1	22	8	1	8	3	1	10	4
Problems with spouse	1	19	6	1	7	3	1	9	3
Problems with relatives	1	11	4	1	6	2	1	7	2
Police problems	1	11	4	1	5	2	1	6	2
Accidents	1	7	3	0	3	1	0	3	1
Job problems	-	3	1	-	1	0	-	1	0
Any alcohol problem	**8**	**54**	**22**	**5**	**37**	**14**	**6**	**39**	**15**
Base	*794*	*341*	*1136*	*4809*	*1822*	*6632*	*5603*	*2164*	*7767*

Table 5.21 Alcohol problems by the number of neurotic disorders and sex

Base: Regular drinkers

Alcohol problem	Women			Men			All adults		
	No neurotic disorder	One disorder	Two or more disorders	No neurotic disorder	One disorder	Two or more disorders	No neurotic disorder	One disorder	Two or more disorders
Percentage with each alcohol problem									
Belligerence	5	10	9	14	19	33	10	14	19
Health problems	1	3	10	5	12	26	3	7	16
Problems with friends	1	3	10	5	11	22	3	7	15
Problems with spouse	1	2	8	4	10	10	3	6	9
Problems with relatives	1	2	3	3	4	18	2	3	9
Police problems	0	0	2	3	8	9	2	4	5
Accidents	0	1	1	2	6	4	1	3	2
Job problems	-	-	-	0	1	4	0	1	2
Any alcohol problem	**6**	**13**	**13**	**20**	**32**	**41**	**14**	**21**	**25**
Base	*2937*	*558*	*81*	*3694*	*438*	*59*	*6632*	*996*	*139*

Table 5.22 Significant odds ratios associated with having an alcohol problem (compared with not having a problem)

		Adjusted OR	95% confidence interval
Alcohol consumption level	Light/Moderate	1.00	....
	Fairly heavy	6.93**	(5.78-8.31)
	Heavy	11.85**	(9.45-14.87)
	Very heavy	23.88**	(18.89-30.21)
Neurotic disorder	No neurotic disorder	1.00	....
	Neurotic disorder	1.93**	(1.58-2.34)
Sex	Male	3.00**	(2.52-3.57)
	Female	1.00	....
Age	16-24	3.96**	(2.78-5.65)
	25-34	2.69**	(1.96-3.69)
	35-44	2.14**	(1.53-2.98)
	45-54	1.41 *	(1.00-1.99)
	55-64	1.00	....
Ethnicity	White	1.00	....
	West Indian or African	0.34 *	(0.14-0.83)
	Asian or Oriental	0.26**	(0.09-0.71)
	Other	2.24 *	(1.02-4.91)
Family unit type	Couple, no children	1.00	....
	Couple & child(ren)	1.12	(0.91-1.39)
	Lone parent & child(ren)	1.98**	(1.34-2.94)
	One person	1.21	(0.94-1.55)
	Adult with parents	1.91**	(1.41-2.59)
	Adult with one parent	1.70**	(1.15-2.52)
Occupation type	Non-manual	1.00	....
	Manual	1.20 *	(1.03-1.40)
Accommodation type	Detached	1.00	....
	Semi-detached	1.30 *	(1.04-1.64)
	Terraced	1.40**	(1.11-1.77)
	Flat or maisonette	1.87**	(1.42-2.46)

Significance: * $p<0.05$ ** $p<0.01$

Factors entered in the model which were not significantly associated with alcohol problems were qualifications, employment status, tenure and locality

Table 5.23   Prevalence of neurotic disorder by type of alcohol problem and sex

Base: Regular drinkers

	Bellige-rence	Health prob-lems	Prob-lems with friends	Prob-lems with spouse	Prob-lems with relatives	Police prob-lems	Acci-dents	Job prob-lems	Any alcohol prob-lem	No alcohol prob-lem	All
	%	%	%	%	%	%	%	%	%	%	%
Women											
Neurotic disorder	28	59	56	55	39	[4]	[4]	[0]	31	17	18
No neurotic disorder	72	41	44	45	61	[8]	[5]	[0]	69	83	82
Base	*215*	*45*	*48*	*35*	*41*	*13*	*10*	*0*	*266*	*3311*	*3576*
Men											
Neurotic disorder	17	28	26	24	21	27	33	[9]	18	10	12
No neurotic disorder	83	72	74	76	79	73	67	[12]	82	90	88
Base	*605*	*250*	*233*	*206*	*142*	*154*	*80*	*21*	*901*	*3290*	*4191*
All adults											
Neurotic disorder	20	32	31	28	25	28	34	[9]	21	14	15
No neurotic disorder	80	68	69	72	75	72	66	[12]	79	86	85
Base	*820*	*295*	*281*	*241*	*183*	*167*	*90*	*21*	*1166*	*6601*	*7767*

Table 5.24   Percentage of adults having an alcohol problem by neurotic disorder, alcohol dependence and sex

Base: Regular drinkers

	Neurotic disorder			No neurotic disorder			All		
	Alcohol dependence	No alcohol dependence	All	Alcohol dependence	No alcohol dependence	All	Alcohol dependence	No alcohol dependence	All
Percentage having an alcohol problem									
Women	87	7	13	73	5	6	79	5	7
Men	90	19	33	85	15	20	86	15	22
All adults	89	12	22	83	10	14	85	10	15
Bases:									
Women	*47*	*592*	*639*	*60*	*2877*	*2937*	*107*	*3469*	*3576*
Men	*96*	*401*	*496*	*276*	*3419*	*3694*	*371*	*3819*	*4191*
All adults	*142*	*993*	*1136*	*336*	*6295*	*6632*	*479*	*7289*	*7767*

Table 5.25   Use of drugs by sex

Drugs taken	Women	Men	All adults
	Percentage taking each drug		
	%	%	%
Cannabis	3	6	5
Stimulants	1	2	1
Amphetamines	0	2	1
Cocaine/crack	0	0	0
Hallucinogens inc. Ecstasy	0	2	1
Hallucinogens/psychedelics	0	1	1
Ecstasy	0	1	1
Hypnotics	1	0	1
Sleeping tablets	0	0	0
Tranquilisers	0	0	0
Other drugs:	0	1	0
Solvents	0	0	0
Opiates	0	0	0
Heroin	-	0	0
Any drug	4	7	5
Base	*4908*	*4833*	*9741*

Informants may have taken more than one type of drug

Table 5.26 Use of drugs by age and sex

Drugs taken	Age					
	16-24	25-34	35-44	45-54	55-64	All ages
Women	*Percentage taking each drug*					
Cannabis	10	3	1	1	0	3
Stimulants	2	1	0	-	0	1
Hallucinogens inc. Ecstasy	1	0	0	-	-	0
Hypnotics	1	1	1	0	1	1
Other drugs	0	0	-	-	-	0
Any drug	**10**	**4**	**2**	**1**	**1**	**4**
Base	*917*	*1221*	*1057*	*929*	*784*	*4908*
Men						
Cannabis	18	8	3	0	0	6
Stimulants	6	2	1	0	-	2
Hallucinogens inc. Ecstasy	7	1	0	-	-	2
Hypnotics	1	1	0	0	0	0
Other drugs	2	0	0	-	0	1
Any drug	**19**	**9**	**4**	**1**	**0**	**7**
Base	*947*	*1219*	*1000*	*915*	*753*	*4833*
All adults						
Cannabis	14	6	2	0	0	5
Stimulants	4	1	0	0	0	1
Hallucinogens inc. Ecstasy	4	1	0	-	-	1
Hypnotics	1	1	1	0	1	1
Other drugs	1	0	0	-	1	0
Any drug	**15**	**6**	**3**	**1**	**1**	**5**
Base	*1864*	*2439*	*2056*	*1844*	*1537*	*9741*

Informants may have taken more than one type of drug

Table 5.27   Use of drugs by sex

Base: Adults who took drugs in the past year which have been used more than 5 times in lifetime where the drug is taken a) without prescription, b) more than prescribed, or c) to get high.

Drug(s) taken	Women	Men	All adults
	Percentage taking each drug		
Cannabis	79	94	89
Stimulants	13	24	20
Amphetamines	12	23	19
Cocaine/crack	3	6	5
Hallucinogens inc. Ecstasy	6	25	18
Hallucinogens/psychedelics	6	17	13
Ecstasy	2	13	10
Hypnotics	21	6	12
Sleeping tablets	10	5	7
Tranquilisers	12	3	6
Other drugs:	3	9	7
Solvents	1	4	3
Opiates	2	3	3
Heroin	-	2	2
Any drug	100	100	100
Base	*177*	*327*	*504*

Informants may have taken more than one type of drug

Table 5.28   Percentage of adults taking each drug type who also took another type of drug

Base : Adults who took drugs in the past year which have been used more than 5 times in lifetime where the drug is taken a) without prescripition, b) more than prescribed or c) to get high

Other drugs taken	Cannabis	Stimulants	Hallucinogens inc. Ecstasy	Hypnotics	Other drugs
	Percentage taking each drug				
Cannabis	*	93	96	35	77
Stimulants	21	*	66	25	62
Hallucinogens inc Ecstasy	20	60	*	21	64
Hypnotics	5	14	13	*	30
Other drugs	6	20	23	17	*
Any other drugs	30	93	96	36	80
Base	*449*	*103*	*92*	*58*	*34*

Table 5.29   Use of drugs (grouped) by CIS-R score (grouped) and sex

Drugs taken	CIS-R score (gouped)						All adults
	0-5	6-11	12-17	18 +	0-11	12+	
Women	*Percentage taking each drug*						
Cannabis only	1	4	3	5	2	4	2
Other drugs only	0 ⎤	1 ⎤	2 ⎤	1 ⎤	1 ⎤	2 ⎤	1 ⎤
Cannabis and other drugs	0 ⎦ 1	1 ⎦ 2	1 ⎦ 2	2 ⎦ 4	0 ⎦ 1	1 ⎦ 3	1 ⎦ 1
Any drug	**2**	**5**	**5**	**9**	**3**	**7**	**4**
Base	*2917*	*1116*	*437*	*437*	*4034*	*874*	*4908*
Men							
Cannabis only	3	6	8	7	4	8	4
Other drugs only	0 ⎤	0 ⎤	1 ⎤	3 ⎤	0 ⎤	2 ⎤	0 ⎤
Cannabis and other drugs	2 ⎦ 2	4 ⎦ 4	6 ⎦ 7	4 ⎦ 7	2 ⎦ 2	5 ⎦ 7	2 ⎦ 3
Any drug	**5**	**10**	**16**	**14**	**6**	**15**	**7**
Base	*3539*	*773*	*265*	*256*	*4312*	*521*	*4833*
All adults							
Cannabis only	2	5	5	6	3	6	3
Other drugs only	0 ⎤	1 ⎤	2 ⎤	2 ⎤	0 ⎤	2 ⎤	1 ⎤
Cannabis and other drugs	1 ⎦ 1	2 ⎦ 2	2 ⎦ 4	3 ⎦ 5	1 ⎦ 2	3 ⎦ 4	1 ⎦ 2
Any drug	**4**	**7**	**9**	**11**	**4**	**10**	**5**
Base	*6456*	*1890*	*702*	*694*	*8346*	*1396*	*9741*

Table 5.30 Use of drugs (grouped) by type of disorder and sex

Drugs taken	Mixed anxiety and depressive disorder	Generalised Anxiety Disorder	Depressive episode	Phobia	Obsessive Compulsive Disorder	Panic	Any neurotic disorder	No neurotic disorder	All
Women	*Percentage taking each drug*								
Cannabis only	4	2	6	6	4	1	4	2	2
Other drugs only	1 ⎤	1 ⎤	4 ⎤	3 ⎤	5 ⎤	- ⎤	1 ⎤	1 ⎤	1 ⎤
Cannabis and other drugs	1 ⎦ 2	2 ⎦ 3	3 ⎦ 7	4 ⎦ 6	1 ⎦ 5	4 ⎦ 4	2 ⎦ 3	0 ⎦ 1	1 ⎦ 1
Any drug	**6**	**4**	**13**	**13**	**10**	**6**	**7**	**3**	**4**
Base	*485*	*251*	*133*	*122*	*100*	*50*	*960*	*3948*	*4908*
Men									
Cannabis only	7	7	6	14	7	17	8	4	4
Other drugs only	2 ⎤	3 ⎤	5 ⎤	6 ⎤	4 ⎤	4 ⎤	2 ⎤	0 ⎤	0 ⎤
Cannabis and other drugs	5 ⎦ 7	6 ⎦ 9	6 ⎦ 11	4 ⎦ 10	1 ⎦ 5	5 ⎦ 8	5 ⎦ 7	2 ⎦ 2	2 ⎦ 3
Any drug	**14**	**16**	**17**	**24**	**12**	**26**	**13**	**6**	**7**
Base	*265*	*188*	*88*	*58*	*57*	*43*	*597*	*4236*	*4833*
All adults									
Cannabis only	5	4	6	9	5	9	6	3	3
Other drugs only	1 ⎤	2 ⎤	4 ⎤	4 ⎤	4 ⎤	2 ⎤	2 ⎤	0 ⎤	1 ⎤
Cannabis and other drugs	2 ⎦ 4	3 ⎦ 5	4 ⎦ 8	4 ⎦ 8	1 ⎦ 5	5 ⎦ 6	3 ⎦ 4	1 ⎦ 1	1 ⎦ 2
Any drug	**9**	**9**	**14**	**16**	**10**	**15**	**10**	**4**	**5**
Base	*750*	*439*	*220*	*180*	*157*	*93*	*1557*	*8184*	*9741*

Table 5.31   Use of drugs (grouped) by the number of neurotic disorders and sex

Drugs taken	Number of neurotic disorders		
	None	One	Two or more
Women	*Percentage taking each type of drug*		
Cannabis only	2	4	3
Other drugs only	1	1	5
Cannabis and			
other drugs	0	1	3
	1	2	8
Any drug	**3**	**6**	**12**
Base	*3948*	*830*	*130*
Men			
Cannabis only	4	8	8
Other drugs only	0	1	8
Cannabis and			
other drugs	2	5	5
	2	6	13
Any drug	**6**	**14**	**21**
Base	*4236*	*519*	*79*
All adults			
Cannabis only	3	6	5
Other drugs only	0	1	6
Cannabis and			
other drugs	1	3	4
	1	4	10
Any drug	**4**	**9**	**15**
Base	*8184*	*1348*	*209*

Table 5.32 Significant odds ratios associated with drug use (compared with no drug use)

		Adjusted OR	95% confidence interval
Neurotic disorder	No neurotic disorder	1.00	....
	Neurotic disorder	2.66**	(2.12-3.34)
Alcohol consumption level	Abstainer/occasional drinker	1.00	....
	Light to moderate	1.62**	(1.14-2.30)
	Fairly heavy	3.95**	(2.66-5.85)
	Heavy	4.75**	(3.02-7.47)
	Very heavy	4.80**	(3.10-7.44)
Sex	Male	1.74**	(1.39-2.18)
	Female	1.00	....
Age	16-24	13.48**	(7.17-25.36)
	25-34	7.05**	(3.77-13.18)
	35-44	3.67**	(1.89-7.13)
	45-54	1.01**	(0.46-2.24)
	55-64	1.00	....
Qualifications	A level or higher	1.00	....
	GCSE/O level	0.74 *	(0.58-0.94)
	Other qualification	0.68 *	(0.47-0.97)
	No qualification	0.64**	(0.48-0.87)
Family unit type	Couple, no children	1.00	....
	Couple & child(ren)	0.58**	(0.40-0.83)
	Lone parent & child(ren)	1.30	(0.79-2.13)
	One person only	2.08**	(1.50-2.89)
	Adult with parents	1.49 *	(1.03-2.16)
	Adult with one parent	1.36	(0.85-2.18)
Employment status	Working full time	1.00	....
	Working part-time	1.77**	(1.29-2.41)
	Unemployed	2.46**	(1.85-3.27)
	Economically inactive	1.62**	(1.14-2.08)
Tenure	Owner-occupier	1.00	....
	Renter	1.62**	(1.29-2.03)

Significance: * $p<0.05$ ** $p<0.01$

Factors entered in the model which were not significantly associated with drug use were: ethnicity, occupation type, accommodation and locality

Table 5.33   Prevalence of neurotic disorder by the use of drugs by sex

Whether had a neurotic disorder	Use of drugs					
	Cannabis only	Other drugs only	Cannabis and other drugs	Any drug	No drugs	All
	%	%	%	%	%	%
Women						
Neurotic disorder	34	36	[14]	37	19	20
No neurotic disorder	66	64	[11]	63	81	80
Base	*116*	*37*	*25*	*177*	*4730*	*4908*
Men						
Neurotic disorder	25	[12]	28	28	11	12
No neurotic disorder	75	[7]	72	72	89	88
Base	*201*	*19*	*107*	*327*	*4507*	*4833*
All adults						
Neurotic disorder	28	45	34	31	15	16
No neurotic disorder	72	55	66	69	85	84
Base	*316*	*155*	*132*	*504*	*9237*	*9741*

Table 5.34   Drug dependence and problems by sex and by age (grouped)

Base: Adults who took drugs in the past year which have been used more than 5 times in lifetime where the drug is taken a) without prescription, b) more than prescribed, or c) to get high

	Sex		Age (grouped)			All adults
	Women	Men	16-24	25-34	35-64	
Percentage with drug dependence	38	43	47	28	46	41
Percentage with a drug problem	20	28	34	17	11	25
Base	*177*	*327*	*272*	*152*	*80*	*504*

Table 5.35   Drug dependence and drug problems by neurotic disorder and sex

Base: Adults who took drugs in the past year which have been used more than 5 times in lifetime where the drug is taken a) without prescription b) more than prescribed or c) to get high

	Neurotic disorder	No neurotic disorder	All
Percentage with drug dependence			
Women	57	26	38
Men	62	35	43
All adults	60	32	41
Percentage with a drug problem			
Women	26	16	20
Men	44	22	28
All adults	36	20	25
Bases			
Women	*66*	*111*	*177*
Men	*92*	*235*	*327*
All adults	*158*	*346*	*504*

Table 5.36   Drug dependence (related to the type(s) of drug taken) and neurotic disorder by the use of drugs

Base: Adults who took drugs in the past year which have been used more than five times in lifetime where the drug is taken a) without prescription b) more than prescribed or c) to get high

Drug dependence related to the type(s) of drug taken, and neurotic disorder	Use of drugs					
	Cannabis only	Other drugs only	Adults who took cannabis and other drugs			Any drug
			Dependence on cannabis	Dependence on non-cannabinoid drugs	Dependence on any drug	
	%	%	%	%	%	%
Dependent	**24**	**57**	**63**	**30**	**74**	**41**
With neurotic disorder	11	34	26	15	30	19
With no neurotic disorder	13	23	37	15	44	22
Not dependent	**76**	**43**	**37**	**70**	**26**	**59**
With neurotic disorder	17	11	8	19	4	13
With no neurotic disorder	59	32	29	51	23	46
Base: Adults who took each type of drug	*316*	*55*	*132*	*132*	*132*	*504*

Table 5.37 Significant odds ratios associated with being drug dependent (compared with not being dependent)

Base: Adults who took drugs in the past year which have been used more than 5 times in lifetime where the drug is taken
a) without prescription b) more than prescribed or c) to get high

		Adjusted O.R	95% C.I
Drug use	Cannabis only	1.00	....
	Other drugs only	4.37**	(2.16-8.83)
	Cannabis and other drugs	9.55**	(5.68-16.03)
Neurotic disorder	No neurotic disorder	1.00	....
	Neurotic disorder	3.41**	(2.10-5.54)
Age	16-24	0.90	(0.46-1.75)
	25-34	0.37**	(0.18-0.76)
	35-64	1.00	....
Ethnicity	White	1.00	....
	West Indian/African	9.06**	(2.04-40.34)
	Asian/Oriental	4.58	(0.75-28.01)
	Other	1.54	(0.12-20.36)
Employment status	Working full-time	1.00	....
	Working part-time	0.95	(0.49-1.83)
	Unemployed	2.18**	(1.24-3.85)
	Economically inactive	1.31	(0.71-2.42)
Occupation type	Non-manual	1.00	....
	Manual	1.70*	(1.07-2.70)

significance: * $p<0.05$ ** $p<0.01$

Factors entered in the model which were not significantly associated with drug dependence were:
alcohol consumption level, sex, family unit type, qualifications, type of accommodation, tenure, and locality

Table 5.38   Significant odds ratios associated with having a drug problem (compared with having no problem)

Base: Adults who took drugs in the past year which have been used more than 5 times in lifetime where drug is taken
a) without prescription b) more than prescribed or c) to get high

		Adjusted O.R	95% C.I
Neurotic disorder	No neurotic disorder	1.00	....
	Neurotic disorder	2.02**	(1.19-3.40)
Drug use	Cannabis only	1.00	....
	Other drugs only	2.01	(0.85-4.75)
	Cannabis & other drugs	10.11**	(5.94-17.22)
Family unit type	Couple, no children	1.00	....
	Couple & child(ren)	0.53	(0.16-1.76)
	Lone parent & child(ren)	1.66	(0.47-5.80)
	One person only	1.05	(0.41-2.66)
	Adult with parents	3.73**	(1.42-9.78)
	Adult with one parent	3.91 *	(1.27-11.99)
Employment status	Working full-time	1.00	....
	Working part-time	0.96	(0.43-2.15)
	Unemployed	2.96**	(1.53-5.72)
	Economically inactive	2.36**	(1.12-4.98)
Tenure	Owner-occupier	1.00	....
	Renter	2.04 *	(1.12-3.74)

significance: *   p<0.05   ** p<0.01

Factors entered in the model which were not significantly associated with drug problems were: alcohol consumption level, sex, age, ethnicity, qualifications, occupation type, accommodation type and locality

Table 5.39   Sex, age, and the number of neurotic disorders by the use of drugs, dependence and problems

	Adults who took drugs					Others	All adults
	Drug dependence	No drug dependence	Drug problem	No drug problem	All adults who took drugs		
	%	%	%	%	%	%	%
Sex							
Female	32	37	27	38	35	51	50
Male	68	63	73	62	65	49	50
Age							
16-24	62	49	73	47	54	17	19
25-34	21	37	20	34	30	25	25
35-44	11	11	4	13	11	22	21
45-54	3	3	3	3	3	20	19
55-64	4	1	0	3	2	16	16
Neurotic disorder							
Neurotic disorder	46	21	45	27	31	15	16
No neurotic disorder	54	79	55	73	69	85	84
Base	*207*	*297*	*127*	*377*	*504*	*9237*	*9741*

Table 5.40 Cigarette smoking by sex: a comparison with the 1993 Health Survey

Cigarette smoking	Psychiatric Morbidity Survey		1993 Health Survey Adults aged 16-64	
	%		%	
Women				
Never regular	51		51	
Ex-regular	18		20	
Light	8		8	
Moderate	13	31	12	30
Heavy	10		9	
Base	*4899*		*6941*	
Men				
Never regular	42		43	
Ex-regular	25		27	
Light	8		7	
Moderate	12	32	10	30
Heavy	12		12	
Base	*4822*		*6298*	
All adults				
Never regular	47		47	
Ex-regular	22		23	
Light	8		8	
Moderate	13	32	12	30
Heavy	11		10	
Base	*9720*		*13239*	

Source: 1993 Health Survey data, OPCS

Cigarette smoking could not be measured for 21 informants on the Psychiatric Morbidity Survey and for 25 informants on the Health Survey.

Table 5.41   Cigarette smoking by age (grouped)

Cigarette smoking	Age (grouped)					All adults
	16-24	25-34	35-44	45-54	55-64	
	%	%	%	%	%	%
Women						
Never regular	53	54	49	48	49	51
Ex-regular	10	14	20	22	26	18
Light	14	8	7	7	5	8
Moderate	17 · 37	13 · 32	12 · 31	11 · 29	12 · 26	13 · 31
Heavy	6	10	13	11	9	10
Base	*916*	*1218*	*1054*	*927*	*783*	*4899*
Men						
Never regular	56	46	41	36	30	42
Ex-regular	7	18	28	35	46	25
Light	14	8	6	4	5	8
Moderate	17 · 37	15 · 36	10 · 31	10 · 29	8 · 24	12 · 32
Heavy	6	13	15	15	11	12
Base	*945*	*1217*	*999*	*913*	*748*	*4822*
All adults						
Never regular	54	50	45	42	40	47
Ex-regular	8	16	24	29	36	22
Light	14	8	6	6	5	8
Moderate	17 · 37	14 · 34	11 · 31	10 · 29	10 · 25	13 · 32
Heavy	6	12	14	13	10	11
Base	*1861*	*2435*	*2053*	*1840*	*1531*	*9720*

Table 5.42   Cigarette smoking by CIS score (grouped) and sex

Cigarette smoking	CIS-score (grouped)						
	0-5	6-11	12-17	18+	0-11	12+	All adults
	%	%	%	%	%	%	%
Women							
Never regular	56	48	43	36	53	39	51
Ex-regular	18	19	19	16	18	18	18
Light	8	8	10	9	8	9	8
Moderate	12 ⎤ 27	14 ⎤ 34	15 ⎤ 38	18 ⎤ 48	12 ⎤ 29	16 ⎤ 43	13 ⎤ 31
Heavy	7 ⎦	11 ⎦	14 ⎦	22 ⎦	8 ⎦	18 ⎦	10 ⎦
Base	*2916*	*1113*	*435*	*435*	*4028*	*870*	*4899*
Men							
Never regular	46	37	29	30	44	29	42
Ex-regular	25	28	22	22	26	22	25
Light	7	7	11	8	7	10	8
Moderate	11 ⎤ 29	14 ⎤ 35	22 ⎤ 50	14 ⎤ 48	12 ⎤ 30	18 ⎤ 49	12 ⎤ 32
Heavy	11 ⎦	14 ⎦	16 ⎦	26 ⎦	11 ⎦	21 ⎦	12 ⎦
Base	*3531*	*772*	*264*	*254*	*4303*	*519*	*4822*
All adults							
Never regular	50	43	38	34	48	36	47
Ex-regular	22	22	20	18	22	19	22
Light	8	8	10	9	8	10	8
Moderate	11 ⎤ 28	14 ⎤ 34	18 ⎤ 42	16 ⎤ 48	12 ⎤ 29	17 ⎤ 45	13 ⎤ 32
Heavy	9 ⎦	12 ⎦	15 ⎦	23 ⎦	10 ⎦	19 ⎦	11 ⎦
Base	*6447*	*1884*	*700*	*689*	*8331*	*1389*	*9720*

Table 5.43 Cigarette smoking by type of neurotic disorder and sex

Cigarette smoking	Type of neurotic disorder								All
	Mixed anxiety and depressive disorder	Generalised Anxiety Disorder	Depressive episode	All phobias	Obsessive-Compulsive Disorder	Panic disorder	Any neurotic disorder	No neurotic disorder	
	%	%	%	%	%	%	%	%	%
Women									
Never regular	42	37	30	43	47	23	40	54	51
Ex-regular	18	16	16	13	12	25	17	18	18
Light	9	10	11	13	9	7	9	8	8
Moderate	16 (39)	17 (48)	20 (53)	12 (44)	18 (42)	19 (52)	16 (43)	12 (28)	13 (31)
Heavy	15	21	23	19	15	26	17	8	10
Base	*483*	*251*	*132*	*121*	*98*	*50*	*956*	*3943*	*4899*
Men									
Never regular	30	27	27	17	33	12	29	44	42
Ex-regular	22	27	13	27	29	29	24	26	25
Light	10	10	12	8	5	13	9	7	8
Moderate	21 (48)	13 (46)	16 (60)	22 (56)	12 (38)	19 (59)	18 (47)	12 (30)	12 (32)
Heavy	17	22	32	26	21	26	20	11	12
Base	*264*	*187*	*88*	*57*	*57*	*43*	*595*	*4227*	*4822*
All adults									
Never regular	38	33	29	34	42	18	36	49	47
Ex-regular	20	20	15	17	18	27	20	22	22
Light	9	10	11	11	8	10	9	8	8
Moderate	18 (42)	16 (47)	18 (56)	15 (48)	16 (40)	19 (55)	17 (44)	12 (29)	13 (32)
Heavy	16	22	26	22	17	26	18	10	11
Base	*748*	*437*	*220*	*178*	*155*	*93*	*1550*	*8170*	*9720*

Cigarette smoking could not be measured for 21 informants

Table 5.44 Cigarette smoking by the number of neurotic disorders and sex

Cigarette smoking	Women			Men			All adults		
	None	One	2 or more	None	One	2 or more	None	One	2 or more
	%	%	%	%	%	%	%	%	%
Never regular	54	41	36	44	30	20	49	37	30
Ex-regular	18	18	13	26	24	22	22	20	16
Light	8	9	10	7	9	12	8	9	11
Moderate	12 (28)	16 (41)	18 (50)	12 (30)	18 (46)	16 (59)	12 (29)	17 (43)	17 (54)
Heavy	8	17	22	11	18	32	10	17	26
Base	*3943*	*826*	*129*	*4227*	*517*	*78*	*8170*	*1343*	*208*

Table 5.45   Significant odds ratios associated with cigarette smoking (compared with not smoking cigarettes)

		Adjusted O.R	95% C.I
Neurotic disorder	No neurotic disorder	1.00	....
	Neurotic disorder	1.60**	(1.41-1.81)
Alcohol consumption level	Abstainer/occasional drinker	1.00	....
	Light to moderate	1.28**	(1.12-1.46)
	Fairly heavy	1.98**	(1.66-2.36)
	Heavy	2.63**	(2.10-3.31)
	Very heavy	2.98**	(2.37-3.76)
Drug use	No drugs taken	1.00	....
	Cannabis only	5.42**	(4.11-7.15)
	Other drugs only	1.69	(0.95-3.00)
	Cannabis & other drugs	10.30**	(6.16-17.21)
Age	16-24	1.42**	(1.15-1.75)
	25-34	1.48**	(1.24-1.76)
	35-44	1.45**	(1.21-1.73)
	45-54	1.33**	(1.12-1.59)
	55-64	1.00	....
Ethnicity	White	1.00	....
	West Indian/African	0.47**	(0.31-1.71)
	Asian/Oriental	0.33**	(0.23-0.49)
	Other	1.41	(0.85-2.34)
Qualifications	A level or higher	1.00	....
	GCSE/O level	1.50**	(1.31-1.71)
	Other	1.65**	(1.39-1.96)
	None	2.44**	(2.12-2.81)
Family unit type	Couple, no children	1.00	....
	Couple & child(ren)	1.05	(0.92-1.19)
	Lone parent & child(ren)	2.03**	(1.64-2.52)
	One person only	1.26**	(1.07-1.48)
	Adult with parents	1.02	(0.82-1.27)
	Adult with one parent	0.97	(0.73-1.30)
Employment status	Working full-time	1.00	....
	Working part-time	0.83**	(0.72-0.95)
	Unemployed	1.30**	(1.10-1.54)
	Economically inactive	0.93**	(0.82-1.06)
Occupation type	Non-manual	1.00	....
	Manual	1.28**	(1.15-1.42)
Accomodation type	Detached	1.00	....
	Semi-detached	1.32**	(1.15-1.53)
	Terraced	1.57**	(1.36-1.82)
	Flat or maisonette	1.61**	(1.35-1.93)
Tenure	Owner-occupier	1.00	....
	Renter	1.62**	(1.44-1.81)

Significance: * p<0.05   ** p < 0.01

Factors entered in the model which were not significantly associated with cigarette smoking were: sex and locality

Table 5.46 Prevalence of neurotic disorder by cigarette smoking and sex

	Never regular	Ex-regular	Light	Moderate	Heavy	All
	%	%	%	%	%	%
Women						
Neurotic disorder	15	19	22	24	34	20
No neurotic disorder	85	81	78	76	66	80
Base	*2491*	*880*	*406*	*632*	*488*	*4899*
Men						
Neurotic disorder	8	12	16	18	20	12
No neurotic disorder	92	88	84	82	80	88
Base	*2048*	*1225*	*363*	*595*	*590*	*4822*
All adults						
Neurotic disorder	12	15	19	21	26	16
No neurotic disorder	88	85	81	79	74	84
Base	*4539*	*2106*	*769*	*1227*	*1079*	*9720*

Table 5.47 Cigarette smoking and drug use by alcohol consumption level and neurotic disorder

Cigarette smoking and drug use	Neurotic disorder				No neurotic disorder				All			
	Abstainer/ Occasional to moderate	Fairly heavy/ heavy	Very heavy	All	Abstainer/ Occasional to moderate	Fairly heavy/ heavy	Very heavy	All	Abstainer/ Occasional to moderate	Fairly heavy/ heavy	Very heavy	All
	%	%	%	%	%	%	%	%	%	%	%	%
Cigarette smoking												
Non-smoker	61	42	26	56	74	62	50	71	72	59	45	68
Light to moderate smoker	24	35	31	26	18	26	25	20	19	27	26	20
Heavy smoker	15	24	44	18	8	13	25	10	9	14	29	11
Drug use	Percentage taking any drug											
All adults	7	20	21	10	3	8	14	4	4	10	16	5
Base	*1204*	*238*	*103*	*1546*	*6324*	*1446*	*377*	*8146*	*7528*	*1684*	*480*	*9692*

Alcohol consumption could not be meausured for 49 infomants, and cigarette smoking could not be measured for 21 informants

Table 5.48 Alcohol consumption level and cigarette smoking by the use of drugs and neurotic disorder

Alcohol consumption level and cigarette smoking	Neurotic disorder			No neurotic disorder			All		
	Took drugs	Others	All	Took drugs	Others	All	Took drugs	Others	All
	%	%	%	%	%	%	%	%	%
Alcohol consumption level									
Abstainer/Occasional to moderate	55	80	78	52	79	78	53	79	78
Fairly heavy to heavy	30	14	15	33	17	18	32	17	17
Very heavy	14	6	7	15	4	5	15	4	5
Cigarette smoking									
Non- smoker	22	59	56	28	73	71	26	71	68
Light to moderate	56	23	26	58	18	20	58	18	20
Heavy	22	18	18	14	10	10	17	11	11
Base	*158*	*1399*	*1557*	*346*	*7838*	*8184*	*504*	*9237*	*9741*

Table 5.49 Alcohol consumption level and drug use by cigarette smoking and neurotic disorder

Alcohol consumption level and drug use	Neurotic disorder				No neurotic disorder				All			
	Non- smoker	Light to moderate smoker	Heavy smoker	All	Non- smoker	Light to moderate smoker	Heavy smoker	All	Non- smoker	Light to moderate smoker	Heavy smoker	All
Alcohol consumption level	%	%	%	%	%	%	%	%	%	%	%	%
Abstainer/Occasional to moderate	86	72	64	78	81	71	65	78	82	71	65	78
Fairly heavy/ heavy	11	20	20	15	15	23	23	18	15	23	22	17
Very heavy	3	8	16	7	3	6	12	5	3	6	13	5
Drug use	*Percentage taking any drug*											
All adults	4	22	12	10	2	13	6	4	2	14	8	5
Base	*861*	*404*	*285*	*1550*	*5784*	*1592*	*794*	*8170*	*6645*	*1996*	*1079*	*9720*

Alcohol consumption could not be measured for 49 informants, and cigarette smoking could not be measured for 21 informants

Table 5.50   Significant odds ratios associated with neurotic disorder (compared with no neurotic disorder)

		Adjusted O.R	95% C.I
Alcohol consumption level	Abstainer/ occasional drinker	1.00	....
	Light to moderate	0.71**	(0.62-0.82)
	Fairly heavy	0.63**	(0.51-0.79)
	Heavy	0.79	(0.59-1.05)
	Very heavy	1.04	(0.79-1.36)
Drug use	No drugs taken	1.00	....
	Cannabis only	1.92**	(1.45-2.54)
	Other drugs only	3.46**	(1.98-6.04)
	Cannabis and other drugs	2.46**	(1.64-3.70)
Cigarette smoking	Non-smoker	1.00	....
	Low	0.95	(0.81-1.10)
	Moderate	1.06	(0.94-1.21)
	Heavy	1.36**	(1.20-1.55)
Sex	Male	1.00	....
	Female	1.63**	(1.42-1.86)
Age	16-24	1.01	(0.79-1.30)
	25-34	1.22	(0.98-1.51)
	35-44	1.46**	(1.17-1.80)
	45-54	1.51**	(1.22-1.86)
	55-64	1.00	....
Family unit type	Couple, no children	1.00	....
	Couple & child(ren)	1.08	(0.92-1.27)
	Lone parent & child(ren)	1.35 *	(1.06-1.73)
	One person only	1.26 *	(1.05-1.53)
	Adult with parents	1.35 *	(0.71-1.24)
	Adult with one parent	1.08	(0.85-1.70)
Employment status	Working full-time	1.00	....
	Working part-time	1.16	(0.98-1.38)
	Unemployed	2.05**	(1.69-2.48)
	Economically inactive	1.60**	(1.36-1.87)
Accommodation type	Detached	1.00	....
	Semi-detached	0.96	(0.81-1.15)
	Terraced	1.16	(0.97-1.39)
	Flat or maisonette	1.24	(1.00-1.54)
Tenure	Owner-occupier	1.00	....
	Renter	1.20**	(1.05-1.38)
Locality	Semi-rural/rural	1.00	....
	Urban	1.21**	(1.06-1.39)

*   p<0.05   ** p<0.01

Factors entered in the model which were not significantly associated with neurotic disorder were: ethnicity, qualifications, and occupation type

6 Adults with a psychotic disorder

6.1 Introduction

In the previous chapters we have looked at adults with neurotic disorders and how they differed from those without neurotic disorders on various characteristics: economic and social circumstances and social functioning. In this chapter, we focus on the relatively small number of adults, forty four in all, who were identified as having a psychotic disorder. (See Appemdix A) Although the socio-demographic characteristics of those with a psychotic disorder were fully described in Report 2, a brief descriptive profile is repeated here as a contextual background.

6.2 Descriptive profile

Adults with a psychotic disorder were equally represented among men and women. About half were aged 16-34 and the largest proportion, 38%, were in the 25-34 age group. Fifty percent of adults with schizophrenia or bipolar affective disorder were married or cohabiting, 30% were single, and 20% were widowed, divorced or separated. Four in five of those who were part of a couple had at least one child.

About a third of the 44 adults with a psychotic disorder had obtained qualifications at A level or at a higher level; a similar proportion were in Social Class I II or III non-manual. In terms of their household characteristics, 59% were living in a terraced house flat or maisonette; and 78% were living in an urban locality.

Because of the relatively small numbers of adults (44) with a psychotic disorder identified from the survey, comparisons with other groups - those with a neurotic disorder (1557)

or those with no psychiatric disorder (8184) - require caution in their interpretation.

6.3 Economic activity

Economic activity among those with a psychotic disorder is significantly different from those with a neurotic disorder or with no psychiatric problems in two main respects. Only four in ten adults with a psychotic disorder were working compared with nearly six in ten of those with a neurotic disorder and 7 in 10 of those unaffected by a mental disorder. Adults with psychosis who were not working were not however different from the other groups in the proportions unemployed; they were, for the most part, economically inactive. One in five described themselves as permanently unable to work (compared with one in fifty among the population with no disorder) and one in ten as retired, presumably on medical grounds. *(Table 6.1)*

The financial consequences of the different patterns of economic activity among those with a psychotic disorder compared with other groups is clearly evident in the survey measures of financial circumstances. In comparison with the sample without a psychiatric disorder, those with psychosis were far more likely to be receiving Income Support, Invalidity Benefit, Sickness Benefit, Disability Living Allowance and Attendance Allowance. The median, weekly, gross, individual income of the group with psychosis was £90 compared with £150 for those without a psychiatric disorder. Although a larger proportion of those with a neurotic than a psychotic disorder were working, their corresponding weekly income was also £90. *(Table 6.2)*

6.4 Activities of Daily Living

Adults with a psychotic illness were similar to those with a neurotic illness in that they were both three times more likely than those without a disorder to have difficulty with at least one activity of daily living. However, the task which caused difficulty among the largest proportion of the psychotic and neurotic groups was different. Among those with psychoses, 22% had difficulty managing money such as budgeting for food or paying bills whereas for the neurotic group, the largest proportion, 18%, had difficulties with practical activities - gardening, decorating, or doing household repairs.

6.5 Stressful life events

There were no significant differences between people with a psychotic disorder and those with a neurotic disorder in terms of the number of stressful life events experienced in the past six months. About two thirds of each group had at least one stressful life event in the past 6 months compared with a half of the sample who had no psychiatric disorder. The extent to which most types of stressful life events were experienced by those with psychotic or with neurotic disorders was also very similar.

6.6 Social functioning

The social functioning of survey respondents was described by various measures or indices: the size of their primary support group, the degree of perceived leisure support, and participation in leisure activities within and outside the home. Adults with a psychotic disorder seemed slightly worse off than those with a neurotic disorder who in turn had less social support than those without a disorder:

- 61% of people with psychosis had a primary support group of less than 9 people compared with 53% of those with a neurotic disorder and 36% of those with neither disorder.

- 54% of people with psychosis felt a moderate or severe lack of social support compared with 45% of people with neurosis and 36% of those with no psychiatric disorder.

In terms of leisure activities, there were no marked differences in participation rates between the psychotic, neurotic and no disorder groups. Any apparent differences can be explained by their different socio-economic and socio-demographic profiles. This can be illustrated with an outdoor and an indoor activity. Those with a psychotic disorder seem more likely than those with no disorder to go to night clubs or discos (28% cf 18%). However, fifty four percent of the sample with a psychotic disorder were aged 16-34 compared with 45% of the no-disorder group. Adults with a psychotic disorder also seemed more likely than others to indulge in hobbies (48% compared with 35%). As we have shown earlier, adults with psychosis are more likely than other groups to be economically inactive, more likely to be living on their own and have smaller numbers of close friends, thus giving the time and opportunity to spend time on their hobbies.

One initially surprising finding in Table 6.6 is that the proportion of people with psychoses who went to clubs and organisations (28%) was larger than the corresponding proportions among those with neuroses (15%), and with no disorder (20%). One would have expected the smallest proportion to have been found among the psychotic group as they appear to have least well developed social networks and social support. However, the results in Table 6.7 may provide the explanation. Ten percent of the adults with psychosis went to a 'club for people with mental health problems' and 5% attended 'a Day Centre for social reasons'. Hardly any of those in the other groups did this.

6.7 Cigarette smoking, alcohol consumption and drug use

Whereas a third of those with a psychotic disorder or a neurotic disorder had never smoked cigarettes, about a half of those with no disorder had never started smoking. Thus, the proportion of smokers among the psychotic and neurotic groups (43% and 44% respectively) was about one and a half times the proportion of smokers among those with no psychiatric disorder, 30%.

Table 6.8 shows that, unlike cigarette consumption, the pattern of alcohol consumption was markedly different between the three groups. Nineteen percent of adults with a psychotic disorder did not drink at all compared with eleven percent of the neurotic sample and seven percent of those without a psychiatric disorder. Even among the drinkers, the proportion of very heavy drinkers among the psy-

chotic group was lower than among the other groups.

The data on drug use, at the bottom of Table 6.8, shows quite clearly, that those with a psychotic disorder were about twice as likely as those with a neurotic disorder to have used cannabis in the past year (16% compared with 9%) who in turn were twice as likely as those with no disorder to have used this drug (9% compared with 4%). The use of drugs such as cocaine, speed, acid, ecstasy, heroin and opium were so rarely used in the population that comparisons between groups are difficult to make.

Table 6.1 Economic activity of adults with (a) a psychotic disorder, (b) a neurotic disorder and (c) no psychiatric disorder

	Adults with a psychotic disorder	Adults with a neurotic disorder	Adults with no psychiatric disorder
	%	%	%
Working	39	56	71
Looking for work	11	11	7
Intending to look, temporarily sick	2	2	2
Permanently unable to work	21	12	2
Retired	10	2	4
Full time education	5	4	4
Keeping house	9	13	10
Other	2	1	1
Base	*44*	*1557*	*8184*

Table 6.2 Financial situation of adults with (a) a psychotic disorder, (b) a neurotic disorder and (c) no psychiatric disorder

	Adults with a psychotic disorder	Adults with a neurotic disorder	All adults surveyed in 1993 for the GHS/Omnibus Surveys*
State Benefits	*Percentage receiving each State Benefit*		
Income Support	31	19	10
Invalidity Pension, Benefit, or allowance	17	9	2
Sickness Benefit	11	3	0
Disability Living Allowance	7	2	2
Attendance Allowance	5	1	-
Base	*44*	*1557*	*13,744*
Personal income	Mid-point of income band		
Median, weekly, gross income	£90	£90	£150
Base	*44*	*1557*	*18,760*

* State Benefits data from GHS; Income data from Omnibus survey

Table 6.3   Difficulties with ADL of adults with (a) a psychotic disorder, (b) a neurotic disorder and (c) no psychiatric disorder

	Adults with a psychotic disorder	Adults with a neurotic disorder	Adults with no psychiatric disorder
	%	%	%
Number of ADL difficulties			
0	60	68	88
1	18	14	8
2	10	7	2
3	2	5	1
4	7	3	0
5+	3	3	0
% with any ADL difficulty	**40**	**32**	**12**
Type of ADL difficulty	*Percentage who have difficulty with each activity*		
Practical activities	17	18	5
Dealing with paperwork	16	12	5
Household activities	16	13	2
Using transport	12	11	2
Managing money	22	10	3
Personal Care	3	7	1
Medical Care	3	2	1
Base	*44*	*1557*	*8184*

Table 6.4 Stressful life events of adults with (a) a psychotic disorder, (b) a neurotic disorder and (c) no psychiatric disorder

	Adults with a psychotic disorder	Adults with a neurotic disorder	Adults with no psychiatric disorder
	%	%	%
Number of stressful life events experienced in past 6 months			
0	37	29	52
1	20	33	31
2	24	22	12
3	9	10	4
4 or more	9	7	1
Any stressful life event	**63**	**71**	**48**
Type of stressful life event	*Percentage of adults experiencing each event in past 6 months*		
Death of other relative	2	19	15
Serious illness of close relative	22	19	12
Seeking work unsuccessfully	16	17	11
Serious problem with close friend	24	21	7
Valuable possessions lost/stolen	16	11	6
Serious personal illness	10	11	4
Breakup of marriage/relationship	9	10	4
Major financial crisis	11	11	4
Made redundant from job	2	6	4
Death of close relative	20	5	3
Problems with police - in court	1	4	1
Base	*44*	*1557*	*8184*

Table 6.5 Size of primary support group and degree of perceived social support for adults with (a) a psychotic disorder (b) a neurotic disorder and (c) no psychiatric disorder

	Adults with a psychotic disorder	Adults with a neurotic disorder	Adults with no psychiatric disorder
	%	%	%
Size of primary support group			
9+	39	48	64
4-8	50	40	31
0-3	11	13	6
Perceived social support			
No lack	46	55	66
Moderate lack	34	28	26
Severe lack	20	17	8
Base	*44*	*1557*	*8184*

Table 6.6   Participation in outdoor and indoor leisure activities for adults with (a) a psychotic disorder, (b) a neurotic disorder, and (c) no psychiatric disorder

Leisure activities	Adults with a psychotic disorder	Adults with a neurotic disorder	Adults with no psychiatric disorder
Out of the home			
	Percentage participating in each activity		
Visiting friends or relatives	70	73	76
Pubs, restaurants	56	61	70
Shopping	56	66	68
Going for a walk, walking the dog	42	49	54
Sports as a participant	32	36	50
Cinema, theatre, concerts	43	38	46
Library	22	21	21
Clubs, organisations	28	15	20
Sports as a spectator	20	14	20
Night clubs, discos	28	16	18
Church	19	13	15
Classes or lectures	11	9	10
Bingo, amusement arcades	8	7	7
Bookmakers, betting & gambling	8	4	5
Political activities	1	2	1
In and around the home			
	Percentage participating in each activity		
TV/radio	80	87	91
Reading books/newspapers	56	66	71
Listening to music	73	67	67
Entertaining friends & relatives	48	51	56
Gardening	30	37	46
Writing letters/telephoning	33	38	36
Hobbies	48	35	34
Games	35	26	31
DIY/car maintenance	19	19	28
Base	*44*	*1557*	*8184*

Table 6.7   Attendance at social, training, or educational centres of adults with (a) a psychotic disorder (b) a neurotic disorder and (c) no psychiatric disorder

	Adults with a psychotic disorder	Adults with a neurotic disorder	Adults with no psychiatric disorder
	Percentage attending each type of centre		
Club for people with mental health problems	10	0	0
Adult Education Centre	7	3	4
Adult Training Centre	5	1	1
Day Centre	5	1	1
Club for people with physical health problems	1	0	0
Base	*44*	*1557*	*8184*

Table 6.8   Use of tobacco, alcohol, and drugs for adults with (a) a psychotic disorder (b) a neurotic disorder and (c) no psychiatric disorder

	Adults with a psychotic disorder	Adults with a neurotic disorder	Adults with no psychiatric disorder
	%	%	%
Cigarette smoking			
Never regular	32	36	49
Ex-regular	26	20	22
Light	11	9	8
Moderate	20 ⎤ 43	17 ⎤ 44	12 ⎤ 30
Heavy	12 ⎦	18 ⎦	10 ⎦
Alcohol consumption level			
Abstainer	19	11	7
Occasional drinker	19	16	12
Light	31	34	39
Moderate	14	17	20
Fairly heavy	10	10	13
Heavy	5	5	5
Very heavy	2	7	5
Drug use			
Cannabis	16	9	4
Stimulants	1	3	1
Hallucinogens inc. Ecstasy	1	2	1
Hypnotics	5	2	0
Other drugs	-	1	0
Any drug	**21**	**10**	**4**
Any drug (excluding cannabis)	**6**	**4**	**1**
Base	*44*	*1557*	*8184*

146

7   Adults with suicidal thoughts

7.1   Introduction

As part of the revised Clinical Interview Schedule, all survey respondents were asked about their experience of depressive symptoms in the seven days prior to interview. Those with significant symptoms in terms of frequency, severity, or duration were also asked questions relating to depressive ideas. Within this context, informants were asked whether they had thought of killing themselves in the past week. Eighty informants, just less than 1% of the total sample, answered 'yes' to this question.

Although the descriptive profile of this group has been presented in Report 2, a brief summary of the profile is presented here which describe the socio-demographic characteristics of these 80 adults with suicidal thoughts.

7.2   Descriptive profile

About two thirds of those who had suicidal thoughts were women, and half were aged 16-34; 28% were aged 16-24. In terms of marital status, just over a third (35%) were married or cohabiting, 36% were single and the remainder (28%) were widowed, divorced or separated. It is therefore not surprising to find that half the sample were either living by themselves or without close relatives, or were lone parents.

A quarter of those who had thoughts about killing themselves were unemployed and about a half were economically inactive; 11% of this group had never worked.

In terms of household characteristics, 58% were renting; the same proportion was living in a terraced house, flat or maisonette. Overall 3 in 4 of those with suicidal thoughts were living in an urban locality.

7.3   Economic activity and financial circumstances

People with suicidal thoughts were distinctly worse off in their economic activity than adults with any neurotic disorder and considerably worse off than those with no psychiatric problems. Two sets of comparisons highlight these difference:

Only about a quarter of adults with suicidal thoughts were working compared with just over a half of those with any neurotic disorder and about three-quarters of those with no psychiatric problem

Among the group who had thoughts of killing themselves, 16% were permanently unable to work, eight times the proportion of people in this position who had no mental disorders.

Table 7.1 also shows that among adults with suicidal thoughts, 13% were still in full-time education compared with 4% of all others. Although those with suicidal thoughts have a larger proportion in the 16-24 age group than either neurotic or the no disorder group (28% compared with 18% and 19% respectively) age alone can not explain this threefold difference. *(Table 7.1)*

The considerable differences in economic activity are also reflected in the financial circumstances of the three groups. Compared with the sample unaffected by psychiatric problems, those with suicidal thoughts were four times more likely to get Income Support (40% compared with 10%) and seven times more likely to be on Invalidity Benefit (14% compared with 2%). Taking into account all sources of income (State Benefits, earned income and unearned income) the median, weekly, gross income of individuals who had thoughts of killing themselves was just less than half that of the no disorder group - £70 compared with £150. *(Table 7.2)*

7.4   Activities of daily living

Thoughts of suicide were not only associated with lack of employment and a relatively low income but were also related to carrying out roles within the home, that is difficulties in carrying out activities of daily living (ADL). Among those with suicidal thoughts, a half had difficulty with at least one activity of daily living compared with a third of those with a neurotic disorder and an eighth of those without a psychiatric disorder.

One in five of those who had thought about killing themselves in the week prior to interview had difficulty with three or more activities. Looking at the types of activities with which they had difficulty, four out of the seven tasks considered were a source of difficulty for about a quarter of this sample: practical activities, household activities, dealing with paperwork and managing money.*(Table 7.3)*

7.5   Stressful life events

Quite clearly, adults with suicidal thoughts were far more likely to experience stressful life events than those with no disorder both in terms of the proportions having any stressful life event and the number of events. Among the potentially suicidal group, 85% had at least one stressful life event in the 6 months prior to interview including 29% with 3 or more events. For the no disorder group, 48% had experienced at least one event including just 5% with 3 or more events. The traumas which those with suicidal thoughts had undergone were fairly evenly spread among many of the different types of events covered by the survey. Between 20-30% of the group with suicidal thoughts said that in the past six months they had experienced at least one of

six stressful life events:

Serious problem with a close friend, neighbour or relative

Suffered from a serious illness, injury or assault

Death of a close family friend or another (not close) relative such as aunt, cousin or grandparent

Separation owing to marital difficulties or breaking off a steady relationship

Seeking worth without success for more than one month

Something valued was lost or stolen

It is also interesting to note that ten percent of the sample who had suicidal thoughts had, in the past six months, problems with the police involving a court appearance, an event which only occurred for one percent of those with no psychiatric disorder. *(Table 7.4)*

7.6   Social support and social functioning

Those who thought of killing themselves in the week prior to interview had a less well developed primary support group and felt a greater lack of social support than all others in the survey. Thirty five percent felt close to three or less people including relatives inside and outside their households and friends. The corresponding figures for the neurotic and no-disorder groups were 13% and 6% respectively. These differences are also reflected in the measure of perceived social support: 43% of the group with suicidal thoughts had a severe lack of perceived social support compared with 17% of those with any neurotic disorder and 8% of those with no psychiatric disorder. *(Table 7.5)*

The relative lack of extensive social networks and social support among a sizeable proportion of those with suicidal thoughts may explain why they were less likely than others to participate in social activities - visiting friends, going to pubs or restaurants, attending clubs or organisations, taking part or being a spectator at sports events, entertaining friends or writing letters to or telephoning people. However, there were no significant differences between those with suicidal thoughts and other survey respondents for activities with a less direct need for extensive social contact - shopping, going for a walk, listening to music, going to the cinema, visiting the library, attending church, or going to classes or lectures. *(Table 7.6)*

A relatively small proportion of respondents, less than 5% of any group, went to social, educational or training centres. *(Table 7.7)*

7.7 Cigarette smoking, alcohol consumption and drug use

Of the three activities, smoking, drinking and drug taking, only the extent of cigarette smoking was significantly different between the group with suicidal thoughts and those with no disorder. Among those with thoughts of killing themselves, 52% were smokers compared with 30% of the no disorder group. Furthermore, among those with suicidal thoughts who smoked, 44% were heavy smokers compared with 33% of smokers with no psychiatric disorder.*(Table 7.8)*

Table 7.1   Economic activity of adults with suicidal thoughts compared with those with a neurotic disorder and those with no psychiatric disorder

	Adults with suicidal thoughts	Adults with a neurotic disorder	Adults with no psychiatric disorder
	%	%	%
Working	27	56	71
Looking for work	17	11	7
Intending to look, temporarily sick	8	2	2
Permanently unable to work	16	12	2
Retired	2	2	4
Full time education	13	4	4
Keeping house	15	13	10
Other	2	1	1
Base	*80*	*1557*	*8184*

Table 7.2   Financial situation of adults with suicidal thoughts compared with those with a neurotic disorder and the general population

	Adults with suicidal thoughts	Adults with a neurotic disorder	All adults surveyed in 1993 for the GHS/Omnibus Surveys*
State Benefits	*Percentage receiving each State Benefit*		
Income Support	40	19	10
Invalidity Pension, Benefit, or allowance	14	9	2
Sickness Benefit	8	3	0
Disability Living Allowance	3	2	2
Attendance Allowance	4	1	-
Base	*80*	*1557*	*13,744*
Personal income	Mid-point of income band		
Median, weekly, gross income	£70	£90	£150
Base	*80*	*1557*	*18,760*

* State Benefits data from GHS; Income data from Omnibus survey

Table 7.3   Difficulties with ADL of adults with suicidal thoughts compared with those with a neurotic disorder and those with no psychiatric disorder

	Adults with suicidal thoughts	Adults with a neurotic disorder	Adults with no psychiatric disorder
	%	%	%
Number of ADL difficulties			
0	50	68	88
1	24	14	8
2	6	7	2
3	4	5	1
4	12	3	0
5+	4	3	0
% with any ADL difficulty	**50**	**32**	**12**
Type of ADL difficulty	*Percentage who have difficulty with each activity*		
Practical activities	24	18	5
Dealing with paperwork	27	12	5
Household activities	23	13	2
Using transport	15	11	2
Managing money	22	10	3
Personal Care	9	7	1
Medical Care	1	2	1
Base	*80*	*1557*	*8184*

Table 7.4   Stressful life events of adults with suicidal thoughts compared with those with a neurotic disorder and those with no psychiatric disorder

	Adults with suicidal thoughts	Adults with a neurotic disorder	Adults with no psychiatric disorder
	%	%	%
Number of stressful life events experienced in past 6 months			
0	15	29	52
1	27	33	31
2	29	22	12
3	14	10	4
4 or more	15	7	1
Any stressful life event	**85**	**71**	**48**
Type of stressful life event	*Percentage of adults experiencing each event in past 6 months*		
Death of other relative	24	19	15
Serious illness of close relative	17	19	12
Seeking work unsuccessfully	20	17	11
Serious problem with close friend	29	21	7
Valuable possessions lost/stolen	20	11	6
Serious personal illness	24	11	4
Breakup of marriage/relationship	21	10	4
Major financial crisis	12	11	4
Made redundant from job	6	6	4
Death of close relative	9	5	3
Problems with police - in court	10	4	1
Base	*80*	*1557*	*8184*

Table 7.5   Size of primary support group and degree of perceived social support for adults with suicidal thoughts compared with those with a neurotic disorder and those with no psychiatric disorder

	Adults with suicidal thoughts	Adults with a neurotic disorder	Adults with no psychiatric disorder
	%	%	%
Size of primary support group			
9+	20	48	64
4-8	45	40	31
0-3	35	13	6
Perceived social support			
No lack	33	55	66
Moderate lack	24	28	26
Severe lack	43	17	8
Base	*80*	*1557*	*8184*

Table 7.6   Participation in leisure activities for adults with suicidal thoughts compared with those with a neurotic disorder and those with no psychiatric disorder

Leisure activities	Adults with suicidal thoughts	Adults with a neurotic disorder	Adults with no psychiatric disorder
Out of the home	*Percentage participating in each activity*		
Visiting friends or relatives	58	73	76
Pubs, restaurants	48	61	70
Shopping	62	66	68
Going for a walk, walking the dog	43	49	54
Sports as a participant	29	36	50
Cinema, theatre, concerts	32	38	46
Library	22	21	21
Clubs, organisations	10	15	20
Sports as a spectator	9	14	20
Night clubs, discos	15	16	18
Church	18	13	15
Classes or lectures	10	9	10
Bingo, amusement arcades	11	7	7
Bookmakers betting & gambling	2	4	5
Political activities	3	2	1
In and around the home	*Percentage participating in each activity*		
TV/radio	75	87	91
Reading books/newspapers	52	66	71
Listening to music	66	67	67
Entertaining friends & relatives	45	51	56
Gardening	31	37	46
Writing letters/telephoning	27	38	36
Hobbies	25	35	34
Games	19	26	31
DIY/car maintenance	15	19	28
Base	*80*	*1557*	*8184*

Table 7.7   Attendance at social, training, or educational centres of adults with suicidal thoughts compared with those with a neurotic disorder and those with no psychiatric disorder

	Adults with suicidal thoughts	Adults with a neurotic disorder	Adults with no psychiatric disorder
	Percentage attending each type of centre		
Club for people with mental health problems	3	0	0
Adult Education Centre	-	3	4
Adult Training Centre	3	1	1
Day Centre	3	1	1
Club for people with physical health problems	1	0	0
Base	*80*	*1557*	*8184*

Table 7.8   Use of tobacco, alcohol, and drugs by those with suicidal thoughts compared with those with a neurotic disorder and those with no psychiatric disorder

	Adults with suicidal thoughts	Adults with a neurotic disorder	Adults with no psychiatric disorder
	%	%	%
Cigarette smoking			
Never regular	31	36	49
Ex-regular	17	20	22
Light	12	9	8
Moderate	17 52	17 44	12 30
Heavy	23	18	10
Alcohol consumption level			
Abstainer	10	11	7
Occasional drinker	13	16	12
Light	28	34	39
Moderate	20	17	20
Fairly heavy	16	10	13
Heavy	7	5	5
Very heavy	7	7	5
Drug use			
Cannabis	5	9	4
Stimulants	1	3	1
Hallucinogens inc. Ecstasy	1	2	1
Hypnotics	5	2	0
Other drugs	2	1	0
Any drug	**12**	**10**	**4**
Any drug (excluding cannabis)	**8**	**4**	**1**
Base	*80*	*1557*	*8184*

Appendix A: Measuring psychiatric morbidity

A1 Identifying neurotic psychopathology

To obtain the prevalence of both symptoms and diagnoses of neurotic psychopathology, the revised version of the Clinical Interview Schedule (CIS–R) was chosen.[1] The CIS–R is made up of 14 sections, each section covering a particular area of neurotic symptoms.

Each section within the interview schedule starts with a variable number of mandatory questions which can be regarded as sift or filter questions. They establish the existence of a particular neurotic symptom in the past month. A positive response to these questions leads the interviewer on to further enquiry giving a more detailed assessment of the symptom in the past week. The symptom is assessed in terms of frequency, duration, severity and time since onset. The informant's responses to these questions determine the score on each section. More frequent and more severe symptoms result in higher scores.

The minimum score on each section is 0, where the symptom was either not present in the past week or was present only in mild degree. The maximum score on each section is 4 (except for the section on Depressive ideas which has a maximum score of 5).

- Summed scores from all 14 sections range between 0 and 57.
- The overall threshold score for significant psychiatric morbidity is 12.
- Symptoms are regarded as significant if they have a score of 2 or more.

The elements contributing to scores on each symptom are shown below:

Fatigue
Scores relate to fatigue or feeling tired or lacking in energy in the past week.
Score one for each of:
- Symptom present on four days or more
- Symptom present for more than three hours in total on any day
- Subject had to push him/herself to get things done on at least one occasion
- Symptom present when subject doing things he/she enjoys or used to enjoy at least once

Sleep problems
Scores relate to problems with getting to sleep, or otherwise, with sleeping more than is usual for the subject in the past week.
Score one for each of:
- Had problems with sleep for four nights or more
- Spent at least 4 hours trying to get to sleep on the night with least sleep
- Spent at least 1 hour trying to get to sleep on the night with least sleep
- Spent three hours or more trying to get to sleep on four nights or more
- Slept for at least 4 hours longer than usual for subject on any night
- Slept for at least 1 hour longer than usual for subject on any night
- Slept for more than three hours longer than usual for subject on four nights or more

Irritability
Scores relate to feelings of irritability, being short-tempered or angry in the past week.
Score one for each of:
- Symptom present for four days or more
- Symptom present for more than one hour on any day
- Wanted to shout at someone (even if subject had not actually shouted)
- Had arguments, rows or quarrels or lost temper with someone and felt it was unjustified on at least one occasion

Worry
Scores relate to subject's experience of worry in the past week, other than worry about physical health.
Score one for each of:
- Symptom present on four or more days
- Has been worrying too much in view of circumstances
- Symptom has been very unpleasant
- Symptom lasted over three hours in total on any day

Depression
Applies to subjects who felt sad, miserable or depressed or unable to enjoy or take an interest in things as much as usual, in the past week. Scores relate to the subject's experience in the past week.
Score one for each of:
- Unable to enjoy or take an interest in things as much as usual

- Symptom present on four days or more
- Symptom lasted for more than three hours in total on any day
- When sad, miserable or depressed subject did not become happier when something nice happened, or when in company

Depressive ideas
Applies to subjects who had a score of 1 for depression. Scores relate to experience in the past week.
Score one for each of:
- Felt guilty or blamed him/herself at least once when things went wrong when it had not been his/her fault
- Felt not as good as other people
- Felt hopeless
- Felt that life isn't worth living
- Thought of killing him/herself

Anxiety
Scores relate to feeling generally anxious, nervous or tense in the past week. These feelings were not the result of a phobia.
Score one for each of:
- Symptom present on four or more days
- Symptom had been very unpleasant
- When anxious, nervous or tense, had one or more of following symptoms:
    heart racing or pounding
    hands sweating or shaking
    feeling dizzy
    difficulty getting breath
    butterflies in stomach
    dry mouth
    nausea or feeling as though he/she wanted to vomit
- Symptom present for more than three hours in total on any one day

Obsessions
Scores relate to the subject's experience of having repetitive unpleasant thoughts or ideas in the past week.
Score one for each of:
- Symptom present on four or more days
- Tried to stop thinking any of these thoughts
- Became upset or annoyed when had these thoughts
- Longest episode of the symptom was $1/4$ hour or longer

Concentration and forgetfulness
Scores relate to the subject's experience of concentration problems and forgetfulness in the past week.
Score one for each of:
- Symptoms present for four days or more
- Could not always concentrate on a TV programme, read a newspaper article or talk to someone

without mind wandering
- Problems with concentration stopped subject from getting on with things he/she used to do or would have liked to do
- Forgot something important

Somatic symptoms
Scores relate to the subject's experience in the past week of any ache, pain or discomfort which was brought on or made worse by feeling low, anxious or stressed.
Score one for each of:
- Symptom present for four days or more
- Symptom lasted more than three hours on any day
- Symptom had been very unpleasant
- Symptom bothered subject when doing something interesting

Compulsions
Scores relate to the subject's experience of doing things over again when subject had already done them in the past week.
Score one for each of:
- Symptom present on four days or more
- Subject tried to stop repeating behaviour
- Symptom made subject upset or annoyed with him/herself
- Repeated behaviour three or more times when it had already been done

Phobias
Scores relate to subject's experience of phobias or avoidance in the past week
Score one for each of:
- Felt nervous/anxious about a situation or thing four or more times
- On occasions when felt anxious, nervous or tense, had one or more of following symptoms:
    heart racing or pounding
    hands sweating or shaking
    feeling dizzy
    difficulty getting breath
    butterflies in stomach
    dry mouth
    nausea or feeling as though he/she wanted to vomit
- Avoided situation or thing at least once because it would have made subject anxious, nervous or tense
- Avoided situation or thing four times or more because it would have made subject anxious, nervous or tense

Worry about physical health
Scores relate to experience of the symptom in the past week.
Score one for each of:
- Symptom present on four days or more
- Subject felt he/she had been worrying too much in view of actual health

- Symptom had been very unpleasant
- Subject could not be distracted by doing something else

Panic

Applies to subjects who felt anxious, nervous or tense in the past week and the scores relate to the resultant feelings of panic, or of collapsing and losing control in the past week.
Score one for each of:
- Symptom experienced once
- Symptom experienced more than once
- Symptom had been very unpleasant or unbearable
- An episode lasted longer than 10 minutes

Any combination of the elements produce the section score.

As well as having certain significant symptoms, other criteria had to be met for a neurotic diagnosis to be obtained. The algorithms for identifying each disorder are shown below.

Algorithms for production of ICD-10 diagnoses of neurosis from the CIS-R ('scores' refer to CIS-R scores)

F32.00 Mild depressive episode without somatic symptoms
1. Symptom duration ≥ 2 weeks

2. *Two or more from:*
- depressed mood
- loss of interest
- fatigue

3. *Two or three from:*
- reduced concentration
- reduced self-esteem
- ideas of guilt
- pessimism about future
- suicidal ideas or acts
- disturbed sleep
- diminished appetite

4. Social impairment

5. *Fewer than four from:*
- lack of normal pleasure /interest
- loss of normal emotional reactivity
- a.m. waking ≥ 2 hours early
- loss of libido

- diurnal variation in mood
- diminished appetite
- loss of ≥ 5% body weight
- psychomotor agitation
- psychomotor retardation

F32.01 Mild depressive episode with somatic symptoms
1. Symptom duration ≥ 2 weeks

2. *Two or more from:*
- depressed mood
- loss of interest
- fatigue

3. *Two or three from:*
- reduced concentration
- reduced self-esteem
- ideas of guilt
- pessimism about future
- suicidal ideas or acts
- disturbed sleep
- diminished appetite

4. Social impairment

5. *Four or more from:*
- lack of normal pleasure /interest
- loss of normal emotional reactivity
- a.m. waking ≥ 2 hours early
- loss of libido
- diurnal variation in mood
- diminished appetite
- loss of ≥5% body weight
- psychomotor agitation
- psychomotor retardation

F32.10 Moderate depressive episode without somatic symptoms
1. Symptom duration ≥2 weeks

2. *Two or more from:*
- depressed mood
- loss of interest
- fatigue

3. *Four or more from:*
- reduced concentration
- reduced self-esteem
- ideas of guilt
- pessimism about future
- suicidal ideas or acts

- disturbed sleep
- diminished appetite

4. Social impairment

5. *Fewer than four* from:

- lack of normal pleasure/interest
- loss of normal emotional reactivity
- a.m. waking ≥ 2 hours early
- loss of libido
- diurnal variation in mood
- diminished appetite
- loss of ≥ 5% body weight
- psychomotor agitation
- psychomotor retardation

F32.11 Moderate depressive episode with somatic symptoms

1. Symptom duration ≥2 weeks

2. *Two or more* from:

- depressed mood
- loss of interest
- fatigue

3. *Four or more* from:

- reduced concentration
- reduced self-esteem
- ideas of guilt
- pessimism about future
- suicidal ideas or acts
- disturbed sleep
- diminished appetite

4. Social impairment

5. *Four or more* from:

- lack of normal pleasure /interest
- loss of normal emotional reactivity
- a.m. waking ≥2 hours early
- loss of libido
- diurnal variation in mood
- diminished appetite
- loss of ≥ 5% body weight
- psychomotor agitation
- psychomotor retardation

F32.2 Severe depressive episode

1. *All three* from:

- depressed mood
- loss of interest
- fatigue

2. *Four or more* from:

- reduced concentration
- reduced self-esteem
- ideas of guilt
- pessimism about future
- suicidal ideas or acts
- disturbed sleep
- diminished appetite

3. Social impairment

4. *Four or more* from:

- lack of normal pleasure /interest
- loss of normal emotional reactivity
- a.m. waking ≥ 2 hours early
- loss of libido
- diurnal variation in mood
- diminished appetite
- loss of ≥ 5% body weight
- psychomotor agitation
- psychomotor retardation

F40.00 Agoraphobia without panic disorder
1. Fear of open spaces and related aspects: crowds, distance from home, travelling alone
2. Social impairment
3. Avoidant behaviour must be prominent feature
4. Overall phobia score ≥ 2
5. No panic attacks

F40.01 Agoraphobia with panic disorder
1. Fear of open spaces and related aspects: crowds, distance from home, travelling alone
2. Social impairment
3. Avoidant behaviour must be prominent feature
4. Overall phobia score ≥ 2
5. Panic disorder (overall panic score ≥ 2)

F40.1 Social phobias
1. Fear of scrutiny by other people: eating or speaking in public etc.
2. Social impairment
3. Avoidant behaviour must be prominent feature
4. Overall phobia score ≥ 2

F40.2 Specific (isolated) phobias
1. Fear of specific situations or things, e.g. animals, insects, heights, blood, flying, etc.
2. Social impairment
3. Avoidant behaviour must be prominent feature
4. Overall phobia score ≥ 2

F41.0 Panic disorder
1. Criteria for phobic disorders not met
2. Recent panic attacks
3. Anxiety-free between attacks
4. Overall panic score ≥ 2

F41.1 Generalised Anxiety Disorder
1. Duration ≥ 6 months
2. Free-floating anxiety
3. Autonomic overactivity
4. Overall anxiety score ≥ 2

F41.2 Mixed anxiety and depressive disorder
1. (Sum of scores for each CIS-R section) ≥ 12
2. Criteria for other categories not met

F42 Obsessive-Compulsive Disorder
1. Duration ≥ 2 weeks
2. At least one act/thought resisted
3. Social impairment
4. Overall scores:
   obsession score=4, or
   compulsion score=4, or
   obsession+compulsion scores ≥6

Those with CIS–R scores of 12 or more, who did not fit the criteria for any of the nine neurotic disorders listed above, were categorised as having mixed anxiety and depressive disorder.

A2 Identifying psychotic psycho-pathology

A sift interview was conducted using an instrument specifically designed for this survey, the psychosis screening questionnaire.[2] Once those with a potential psychotic disorder had been identified, Schizophrenia and other functional psychoses were derived from SCAN[3] interviews by clinicians. A diagnosis of 'psychosis unspecified' was also made on the basis of data collected by OPCS interviewers when clinical assessments could not be made.

A3 Obtaining the classification system of different disorders

The survey identified three psychotic and nine specific neurotic disorders from SCAN and CIS–R results, based on ICD–10 diagnostic criteria.[4]

The psychotic disorders were combined in one group and the neurotic disorders were grouped into 6 diagnostic classes for most analysis. The derivation of the various disorders and the way in which the information was analysed is shown below.

Although it was possible for individuals to have more than one disorder, in Report 1 each individual was classified according to their most severe, or primary disorder. The hierarchy used to determine the primary disorder is shown below.

Primary disorder hierarchy used for prevalence estimates in Report 1 (disorders listed in descending order of severity)

A Any psychotic disorder

B Neurotic disorders as follows:

1 severe depressive episode
2 moderate depressive episode
3 panic disorder
4 Obsessive–Compulsive Disorder (OCD)
5 mild depressive episode
6 social phobia
7 agoraphobia
8 Generalised Anxiety Disorder (GAD)
9 specific isolated phobia
10 mixed anxiety and depressive disorder

Once the most severe disorder had been identified, some of the categories were collapsed such that severe, moderate and mild depressive episode were grouped under 'depressive episode' and social phobia, agoraphobia and specific isolated phobia were described collectively as 'phobias'.

Notes and references

1. Lewis, G. and Pelosi, A. J., *Manual of the Revised Clinical Interview Schedule, (CIS–R)*, June 1990, Institute of Psychiatry.

    Lewis, G., Pelosi, A.J., Araya, R.C. and Dunn, G., (1992) Measuring psychiatric disorder in the community: a standardized assessment for use by lay interviewers, *Psychological Medicine*, 22, 465–486

2. Bebbington, P.E., and Nayani, T (1995). The psychosis screening questionnaire. *International Journal of Methods in Psychiatric Research*. Volume 5:11–19

3. *Schedules for Clinical Assessment in Neuropsychiatry*, 1992, WHO, Division of Mental Health, Geneva

4. *WHO, The ICD–10 Classification of Mental and Behavioural Disorders: Diagnostic Criteria for Research*: 1993, WHO, Geneva.

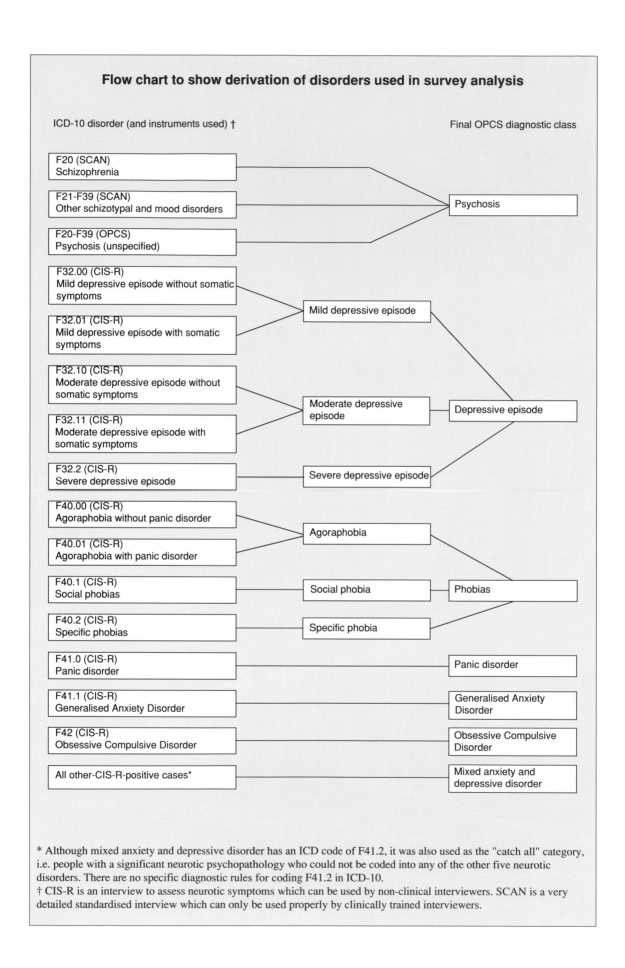

Appendix B Multiple logistic regression (MLR) and Odds Ratios (OR)

B1 Interpretation of Odds Ratios

Chapters 1 to 5 of this report use logistic regression analysis to provide a measure of the effect of having a neurotic disorder on, for example, not working. Unlike many of the crosstabulations presented elsewhere in the report, MLR estimates the effect of a neurotic disorder while controlling for the confounding effect of other variables in the analysis. A forward stepwise method of logistic regression was used. The dependent variable was dichotomous, indicating the presence or absence of a particular behaviour or state. All variables were categorical.

Logistic regression produces an estimate of the probability of an event occurring when an individual is in a particular category of a sociodemographic variable compared to a reference category of that variable. The odds of the event occurring are defined as the ratio of the probability of the event occurring compared with its absence. If the probability of an event is p, the odds are p/(1-p). The factor by which the odds of an event differ for people in a particular category compared with those in the reference category is shown by the Adjusted Odds Ratio (OR). The OR controls for the possible confounding effects of other

variables in the statistical model, eg. sex, age and employment status. To determine whether this increased odds of the event occurring are due to chance rather than to the effect of the variable, the confidence interval associated with the odds ratio is calculated.

B2 Confidence intervals around an Odds Ratio

In Table 1.7, for example, the first odds ratio of 1.52 is shown with a confidence interval from 1.34 to 1.74, indicating that the 'true' (i.e., population) OR is 95% likely to lie between these two values. If the confidence interval does not include 1.00 then the OR is likely to be significantly different from the reference category.

B3 Significance

It is stated in the text of the report that some odds ratios are "significant". This indicates that it is unlikely that an odds ratio of this magnitude would be found due to chance alone. Specifically, the likelihood that the OR shows an effect simply by chance is less than 5%. This is conventionally assumed to be infrequent enough to discount chance as an explanation for the finding.

Glossary of survey definitions and terms

Activities of Daily Living

The seven area of functioning covered by the survey were:

- **Personal care** such as dressing, bathing, washing, or using the toilet.

- **Using transport** to get out and about.

- **Medical care** such as taking medicines or pills, having injections or changes of dressing.

- **Household activities** such as preparing meals, shopping, laundry and housework.

- **Practical activities** such as gardening, decorating or doing household repairs.

- **Dealing with paperwork**, such as writing letters, sending cards or filling in forms.

- **Managing money** such as budgeting for food or paying bills.

Respondents were asked whether they had difficulty with each task. Apart from the responses, 'Yes' and 'No', there was also a 'Does Not Apply' category which was used when the activity was not in the daily repertoire of behaviours of the subject. Care was taken that if the activity was not carried out because of a physical or mental health problem, the subject was deemed to have difficulty in carrying out the task.

Adults
In this survey adults were defined as persons aged 16 or over and less than aged 65.

Alcohol consumption
The final classification of alcohol consumption required the amalgamation of detailed information on what alcohol was drunk and the frequency of intake converted into units. The several stages involved in this process were:

1. Establishing how often the subject had the following drinks:

- **Shandy** (excluding bottles or cans)

- **Beer, lager, stout or cider**

- **Spirits or liqueurs** (eg. gin, whisky, rum, brandy, vodka, avocaat)

- **Wine** (including Babycham and champagne)

- **Any other alcoholic drink**

2. For any drink taken in the last year, how much was usually drunk on any one day.

3. Converting measures (pints, cans, singles, glasses) into units.

4. Taking account of the different evaluation of units of alcohol for women and men .

The final classification of weekly alcohol consumption rating was:

- **Abstainer**

- **Occasional** - Men (<1); Women (<1)

- **Light** - Men (1-10); Women (1-7)

- **Moderate** - Men (11-21); Women (8-14)

- **Fairly heavy** - Men (22-35); Women (15-25)

- **Heavy** - Men (36-50); Women (26-35)

- **Very heavy** - Men (51+); Women (36+)

Alcohol dependence
This was derived from responses to a self-completion questionnaire asked of all survey respondents. Individuals were classified as alcohol dependent if they had three or more positive responses to the following twelve statements.

Loss of control

1. Once I started drinking it was difficult for me to stop before I became completely drunk

2. I sometimes kept on drinking after I had promised myself not to.

3. I deliberately tried to cut down or stop drinking, but I was unable to do so.

4. Sometimes I have needed a drink so badly that I could not think of anything else.

Symptomatic behaviour

5. I have skipped a number of regular meals while drinking

6. I have often had an alcoholic drink the first thing when I got up in the morning.

7. I have had a strong drink in the morning to get over the previous night's drinking

8. I have woken up the next day not being able to remember some of the things I had done while drinking.

9. My hand shook a lot in the morning after drinking.

10. I need more alcohol than I used to get the same effect as before.

11. Sometimes I have woken up during the night or early morning sweating all over because of drinking.

Binge Drinking

12. I have stayed drunk for several days at a time.

Antipsychotic drugs

These are also known as 'neuroleptics'. In the short term they are used to quieten disturbed patients whatever the underlying psychopathology. See Depot Injections

Cigarette smoking

Questions on cigarette smoking were taken from the General Household Survey. For those who did smoke the average number of cigarettes smoked per day was calculated from answers to questions on the number of cigarettes usually smoked on weekdays and on weekends. The final classification did not take account of the tar level of cigarettes, only the quantity smoked:

- **Light smoker** - less than 10 a day

- **Moderate smoker** - more than 10 but less than 20 a day

- **Heavy smoker** - at least 20 a day

- **Ex-regular smoker**

- **Never a regular smoker**

Depot injections

When antipsychotic medication is given by injections on a monthly basis, these are sometimes termed depot injections.

Drug dependence

This was derived from responses to a self-completion questionnaire asked of all survey respondents. An individual was classified as drug dependent if they had a positive response to any of the following five questions in relation to the 10 drugs listed in the box below. A prerequisite was that the drug(s) must have been taken either without a prescription, more than was prescribed for the subject, or to get high.

1. Sleeping Pills, Barbiturates, Sedatives, Downers, Seconal

2. Tranquillisers, Valium, Librium

3. Cannabis, Marijuana, Hash, Dope, Grass, Ganja, Kif

4. Amphetamines, Speed, Uppers, Stimulants, Qat

5. Cocaine, Coke, Crack

6. Heroin, Smack

7. Opiates other than herion: Demerol, Morphine, Methadone, Darvon,Opium, DF118

8. Psychedelics, Hallucinogens: LSD, Mescaline, Acid, Peyote, Psylocybin (Magic) mushrooms

9. Ecstasy

10. Solvents, inhalants, glue, amyl nitrate

1. Have you ever used any one of these drugs every day for two weeks or more in the past twelve months?

2. In the past twelve months have you used any one of these drugs to the extent that you felt like you needed it or were dependent on it?

3. In the past twelve months, have you tried to cut down on any drugs but found you could not do it?

4. In the past twelve months did you find that you needed larger amounts of these drugs to get an

163

effect, or that you could no longer get high on the amount you used to use?

5. In the past twelve months have you had withdrawal symptoms such as feeling sick because you stopped or cut down on any of these drugs?

Drug use
Information was initially collected on the use of particular groups of drugs. This was subsumed under more general headings for the purpose of analysis.

- **Cannabis**

- **Stimulants** (cocaine and speed)

- **Hallucinogens** (acid and Ecstasy)

- **Hypnotics** (barbiturates, sedatives, tranquillisers, valium, librium, etc)

- **Other** - heroin, opium, solvents

A subject was classified as having used drugs in the past year if he/she had taken any of these drugs in the past 12 months either without a prescription, more than was prescribed, or to get high, and had taken the drug more than five times in his/her life.

Economic activity
The questions used to measure economic activity were taken from those regularly asked in the General Household Survey. All adults are place into one of eight categories:

- **Working** - having done paid work in the seven days ending the Sunday before the interview, either as an employee or self-employed, including those were not actually at work but had a job they were away from.

- **Looking for work**

- **Intending to look for work** but prevented by temporary, ill-health, sickness or injury

- **Going to school or college full-time** - only used for persons aged 16-49.

- **Permanently unable to work** due to long-term sickness or disability - for women, only used if aged 16-59

- **Retired** - used only if stopped work at the aged of 50 or over

- **Looking after the home or family**

- **Other** - doing something else

Educational level
Educational level was based on the highest educational qualification obtained and was grouped as follows:

Degree (or degree level qualification)

Teaching, HND, Nursing
    Teaching qualification
    HNC/HND, BEC/TEC Higher, BTEC
Higher
    City and Guilds Full Technological
    Certificate
    Nursing qualifications:
    (SRN,SCM,RGN,RM,RHV,
    Midwife)

A level
    GCE A-levels/SCE higher
    ONC/OND/BEC/TEC/not higher
    City and Guilds Advanced/Final level
O level
    GCE O-level (grades A-C if after 1975)
    GCSE (grades A-C)
    CSE (grade 1)
    SCE Ordinary (bands A-C)
    Standard grade (levels 1-3)
    SLC Lower SUPE Lower or Ordinary
    School certificate or Matric
    City and Guilds Craft/Ordinary level

GCSE/CSE
    GCE O-level (grades D-E if after 1975)
    GCSE (grades D-G)
    CSE (grades 2-5)
    SCE Ordinary (bands D-E)
    Standard grade (levels 4-5)
    Clerical or commercial qualifications
    Apprenticeship
    Other qualifications

No qualifications
    CSE ungraded
    No qualifications

Employment status
Four types of employment status were identified: working full time, working part time, unemployed and economically inactive.

Working adults
The two categories of working adults include persons who did any work for pay or profit in the week ending the last Sunday prior to interview, even if it was for as little as one hour, including Saturday jobs and casual work (e.g. babysitting, running a mail order club).

Self-employed persons were considered to be working if they worked in their own business, professional practice, or farm for the purpose of making a profit, or even if the enterprise was failing to make a profit or just being set up.

The unpaid 'family worker' (e.g., a wife doing her husband's accounts or helping with the farm or business) was included as working if the work contributed directly to a business, farm or family practice owned or operated by a related member of the same household. (Although the individual concerned may have received no pay or profit, her contribution to the business profit counted as paid work.) This only applied when the business was owned or operated by a member of the same household.

Anyone on a Government scheme which was employer based was also 'working last week'.

Informants' definitions dictated whether they felt they were working full time or part time.

Unemployed adults
This category included those who were waiting to take up a job that had already been obtained, those who were looking for work, and people who intended to look for work but were prevented by temporary ill-health, sickness or injury. 'Temporary' was defined by the informant.

Economically inactive
This category comprised five main categories of people:

'Going to school or college' only applied to people who were under 50 years of age. The category included people following full-time educational courses at school or at further education establishments (colleges, university, etc). It included all school children (16 years and over).

During vacations, students were treated as 'going to school or college' even where their return to college was dependent on passing a set of exams. If however, they were having a break from full-time education, i.e. they were taking a year out, they were not counted as being in full-time education.

'Permanently unable to work because of long-term sickness or disability' only applied to those under state retirement age, ie to men aged 16 to 64 and to women aged 16 to 59. 'Permanently' and 'long-term' were defined by the informant.

'Retired' only applied to those who retired from their full-time occupation at age 50 or over and were not seeking further employment of any kind.

'Looking after the home or family' covered anyone who was mainly involved in domestic duties, provided this person had not already been coded in an earlier category.

'Doing something else' included anyone for whom the earlier categories were inappropriate.

Ethnicity
Household members were classified into nine groups by the person answering Schedule A.

White	White
Black - Caribbean	
Black - African	West Indian/African
Black - Other	
Indian	
Pakistani	Asian/Oriental
Bangladeshi	
Chinese	
None of these	Other

For analysis purpose these nine groups were subsumed under 4 headings: White, West Indian/African, Asian/Oriental and Other.

Family unit
In order to classify the relationships of the subject to other members of the households, the household members were divided into family units.

Subjects were assigned to a family unit depending on whether they were or ever had been married, and whether they (or their partners) had any children living with them.

A 'child' was defined for family unit purposes as an adult who lives with one or two parents, provided he or she has never been married and has no child of his or her own in the household.

For example, a household containing three women, a grandmother, mother and child would contain two family units with the mother and child being in one unit, and the grandmother being in another. Hence family units can consist of:

- A married or cohabiting couple or a lone parent with their children

- Other married or cohabiting couples

- An adult who has previously been married. If the

adult is now living with parents, the parents are treated as being in a separate family unit

- An adult who does not live with either a spouse, partner, child or parent. This can include adults who live with siblings or with other unrelated people, e.g. flatmates.

Family unit type
Each informant's family unit was classified into one of six family unit types:

'Couple no children' included a married or cohabiting couple without children.

'Couple with child' comprised a married or cohabiting couple with at least one child from their liaison or any previous relationship.

'Lone parent' describes both men and women (who may be single, widowed, divorced or separated) living with at least one child. The subject in this case could be a divorced man looking after his 12 year-old son or a 55 year-old widow looking after a 35 year-old, daughter who had never married and had no children of her own.

'One person' describes the family unit type and does not necessarily mean living alone. It includes people living alone but includes one person living with a sister, or the grandmother who is living with her daughter and her family. It also includes adults living with unrelated people in shared houses, e.g. flatmates.

'Adult living with parents' describes a family unit which has the same members as 'couple with child' but in this case it is the adult son or daughter who is the subject. It includes a 20 year old unmarried student living at home with married or cohabiting parents, and a 62 year old single woman caring for her elderly parents.

'Adult living with lone parent' covers the same situations as above except that there is one and not two parents in the household.

Household
The standard definition used in most surveys carried out by OPCS Social Survey Division, and comparable with the 1991 Census definition of a household, was used in this survey. A household is defined as a single person or group of people who have the accommodation as their only or main residence and who either share one meal a day or share the living accommodation. (See E McCrossan *A Handbook for interviewers*. HMSO: London 1985.)

Locality
Interviewers coded their opinion of whether the sampled address was in an urban, semi-rural or rural area.

Marital status
Informants were categorised according to their own perception of marital status. Married and cohabiting took priority over other categories. Cohabiting included anyone living together with their partner as a couple.

Perceived social support
The level of social support which informants reported was based on responses to the following 7 statements. Respondents could say that each statement was not true, partly true or certainly true.

There are people I know – amongst my family or friends – who...

1. do things to make me happy
2. make me feel loved
3. can be relied on no matter what happens
4. would see that I am taken care of if I needed to be
5. accept me just as I am
6. make me feel an important part of their lives
7. give me support and encouragement

Each response of not true scored 1, partly true scored 2 and certainly true scored 3; individuals therefore had a total score of between 7 and 21.

Social support was classified as:

> severe lack (scores 7 to 17)
> moderate lack (scores 18 to 20)
> no lack (score 21)

Physical complaints
Informants were asked 'Do you have any long-standing illness, disability or infirmity? By long-standing I mean anything that has troubled you over a period of time or that is likely to affect you over a period of time?'

Those that answered yes to this question were then asked 'What is the matter with you?'; interviewers were asked to try and obtain a medical diagnosis, or to establish the main symptoms. From these responses, illnesses were coded to the site or system of the body that was affected, using a classification system that roughly corresponded to the chapter headings of the International Classification of Diseases (ICD–10). Some of the illnesses identified were mental illnesses and these were excluded from the classification of physical illness. Physical illness did, however, include physical disabilities and sensory complaints such as eyesight and hearing problems.

Primary support group

The size of the individual's primary support group was calculated as a measure of the extent of their social networks. In the survey, data were collected about the size of three groups of people:

The **number of adults who lived with the respondent** that they felt close to

The **number of relatives who did not live with the respondent** that they felt close to

The **number of friends or acquaintances who did not live with the respondent** that would be described as close or good friends

The total number of close friends and relatives were regarded as the individual's primary support group. For the purposes of analysis, the total number in the primary support group was categorised into: 3 or fewer, 4-8, and 9 or more.

Psychiatric morbidity

The expression psychiatric morbidity refers to the degree or extent of the prevalence of mental health problems within a defined area.

Region

When the survey was carried out there were 14 Regional Health authorities in England. These were the basis for stratified sampling and have been retained for purposes of analysis. Scotland and Wales were treated as two distinct areas.

Social class

Based on the Registrar General's 1991 *Standard Occupational Classification,* Volume 3 OPCS, HMSO: London social class was ascribed on the basis of the following priorities:

Firstly, social class was based on the informant's own occupation, unless the informant was a married or cohabiting woman. In such cases, the spouse or partner's occupation was used. The exception is where the spouse or partner had never worked, in which case the woman's own occupation was used.

Secondly, social class was based on the informant's (or spouse's) current occupation or, if the informant (or spouse) was unemployed or economically inactive at the time of interview but had previously worked, social class was based on the most recent previous occupation.

The classification used in the tables is as follows:

Descriptive definition	Social class
Professional	I
Intermediate occupations	II
Skilled occupations — non-manual	III NM
Skilled occupations — manual	III M
Partly-skilled	IV
Unskilled occupations	V
Armed Forces	

Social class was not determined where the subject (and spouse) had never worked, or if the subject was a full-time student or where occupation was inadequately described.

Stressful life events

Responses of 'yes' to any of the following 11 questions identified a recent stressful life event.

In the past 6 months...

1. have you yourself suffered from a serious illness, injury or an assault?

2. has a serious illness, injury or an assault happened to a close relative?

3. has a parent, spouse (or partner), child, brother or sister of yours died?

4. has a close family friend or another relative died, such as an aunt, cousin or grandparent?

5. have you had a separation due to marital difficulties or broken off a steady relationship?

6. have you had a serious problem with a close friend, neighbour or relative?

7. were you made redundant or sacked from your job?

8. were you seeking work without success for more than one month?

9. did you have a major financial crisis, such as losing the equivalent of 3 months income?

10. did you have problems with the police involving a court appearance?

11. was something you valued lost or stolen?

Informants were classified according to the number of stressful life events they had experienced in the last 6 months.

Tenure

Four tenure categories were created:

'Owned outright' means bought without mortgage or loan or with a mortgage or loan which has been paid off.

'Owned with mortgage' includes co-ownership and shared ownership schemes.

'Rent from LA/HA' means rented from local authorities, New Town corporations or commissions or Scottish Homes, and housing associations which include co-operatives and property owned by charitable trusts.

'Rent from other source' includes rent from organisations (property company, employer or other organisation) and from individuals (relative, friend, employer or other individual).

Printed in the United Kingdom for HMSO.
Dd.0301904, 12/95, C20, 3400, 5673, 340649.